VGM Opportunities Series

OPPORTUNITIES IN
MODELING CAREERS

Susan Wood Gearhart

Foreword by
Shirley Hamilton
Shirley Hamilton, Inc.
Talent Representation

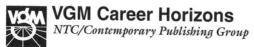

VGM Career Horizons
NTC/Contemporary Publishing Group

Library of Congress Cataloging-in-Publication Data

Gearhart, Susan Wood.
    Opportunities in modeling careers / Susan Wood Gearhart ;
foreword by Shirley Hamilton. — Rev. ed.
      p.   cm. — (VGM opportunies series)
    Includes bibliographical references.
    ISBN 0-8442-1753-0 (cloth). — ISBN 0-8442-1754-9 (pbk.)
    1. Models (Persons)—Vocational guidance. I. Title. II. Title:
Modeling careers. III. Series.
HD6073.M77G43   1999
796.9'2'02373—dc21
                                      98-46530
                                        CIP

Published by VGM Career Horizons
A division of NTC/Contemporary Publishing Group, Inc.
4255 West Touhy Avenue, Lincolnwood (Chicago), Illinois 60646-1975 U.S.A.
Copyright © 1999 by NTC/Contemporary Publishing Group, Inc.
All rights reserved. No part of this book may be reproduced, stored in a retrieval
system, or transmitted in any form or by any means, electronic, mechanical,
photocopying, recording, or otherwise, without the prior permission of NTC/
Contemporary Publishing Group, Inc.
Printed in the United States of America
International Standard Book Number: 0-8442-1753-0 (cloth)
                                           0-8442-1754-9 (paper)

99 00 01 02 03 04 MV 18 17 16 15 14 13 12 11 10 9 8 7 6 5 4 3 2 1

DEDICATION

To Marguerite S. and Wm. Barker Wood,
Gabrielle, Jennifer, Ted, and Finn.

CONTENTS

1. Who Are the Professional Models? 1

Artists' models. Illustrators' models. Promotional models. Garment or fit models. Photographers' models. Runway models and fashion-show work. Male models. Television models. Video models.

2. Attributes Needed for Modeling 20

Looks and attitude. Physical qualifications for high fashion. Qualifications for all models. Qualifications for male models. Qualifications for child models. Qualifications for television models.

3. Breaking into Modeling 36

Are you model material? The beauty contest. Heading for the big agencies. Breaking into television modeling.

ABOUT THE AUTHOR

Susan Wood Gearhart is a professional model, dancer, and freelance writer and editor. She graduated from City University of New York and attended Hiram College, Juilliard School of Music, and the Preibar Academy in Berlin, Germany. She has worked as a professional model since her teens and has covered the field from artist's model to television to runway work. She has modeled for a wide variety of products, from cosmetics to bathing suits, and has made a career of freelance, agency, part-time, and full-time jobs.

FOREWORD

This book is a "must read" for every potential and professional model.

Ms. Gearhart has a knack for getting to the most important, yet usually overlooked, advice that any of us within the industry could offer.

She gives the reader a balanced assessment of a potentially unbalanced business. Her emphasis on hard work and commitment to realistic goals is a very needed message in today's fashion market. An industry that is built on such amorphous ideas as beauty, style, imagination, and impulse may be glamorous to the consumer, but it takes talented people to keep their feet on the ground while portraying an *image* of one with their head in the clouds. Ms. Gearhart also reminds us of a realistic evaluation of ourselves. After all, "popularity must not be confused with possible modeling qualifications."

The major idea you, the reader, will remember—long after you have read this book—is a sense of reality within the business of fantasy. The fashion model is an actor in every sense. You will be portraying a character to your public, whether that character be sultry, classic, sporty, or comic.

Ms. Gearhart reminds us that in fashion, *image* is our business. As a business it must be approached with the same realistic goals we would set in any other career—but, we never forget that fashion is also to be enjoyed.

Shirley Hamilton
Shirley Hamilton Inc.
Talent Representation

PREFACE

Advertising—with the help of masses of people who want to identify with status products—has brought modeling to an all-time celebrity level. For the first time we are experiencing a radical change in this profession as millions of wanna-be models reach for the chance to be discovered and become rich and/or famous. Today it is so desirous to have power money, that our youths look for the get-rich-as-fast-as-you-can path. Few, very few, are truly suited to this profession. It is a career of hard work, discipline, and level-headedness in a world made up of illusionary costumes, hype, and fantasy.

The critical facts are that you must be all of the physical "look" currently in vogue and unique enough to stay on top while thousands covet your job as a Cinderella success story. Though agencies practically bar their doors against the millions of prospective auditioners, the hordes of wanna-bes keep swelling. A recent estimate by one of the top agents in New York City is that one in ten thousand of the hopefuls joins an agency.

I would never discourage anyone from this profession, but we must be realistic. There is a great deal of competition out there, but if you are well prepared, you may be able to find modeling jobs from catalog work to television commercials that come with excellent salaries. Modeling can and often does entail part-time jobs such as a lone TV commercial. But in the grand scheme of things, when this single job pays you $30,000, that's pretty good! As you weigh the many possibilities and your potential to accomplish your goals, arm yourself with all the practical information about the field that you can find and then proceed.

My personal opinion is always to spend the least amount of money you can to find out if this career is for you. Line up for the open call at every good agent's door and hear what he or she has to tell you. Agents are there to make money, have the expertise to help you, and are the first line of this profession. If you are rejected and believe your potential has been overlooked, simply go to another agency's open call. Good luck!

ACKNOWLEDGMENTS

My gratitude and appreciation are extended to the following for their kindness, help, and time: Gabrielle Marguerite Gearhart, model; Joe Hunter of Ford Men, Ford Models, Inc.; Penelope Rudnikoff of Penelope Professional Modelling School and Agency Ltd., Toronto, Canada; Marsha Hall, model; Debbie Balla and Mendy Brannon, *Teen Magazine;* Sean Smith, photographer; Sadie and Tyson; Alisa Allen of Ford Models, Inc., New York City; Gary Bertalovitz, president, and Ken Metz of McDonald/Richards Agency; Barbara W. Donner, former editor, National Textbook Company; Daniela Guggenheim; Nicole Smith; Daisy Chung and Sandra Reith of Sutherland Models, Toronto, Canada.

INTRODUCTION

Recently so much attention has been given to models and their lifestyles that they have become public curiosities. A profession that relies solely on looks rather than ability or talent is a unique phenomenon. Societal demands are such that youth and beauty are articles of admiration and are of great material worth. A product is made of the model, and as such it must be new, nearly unattainable, and expensive. We have wrapped the profession in packaging so difficult to acquire, that it now demands its own place. No wonder modeling is looking more than ever like winning the lottery. You just may become a millionaire first by being the sought-after "look of the moment," and then by being clever enough to make that moment last as long as you can.

Although that illusive and desired look has changed dramatically throughout the centuries, beauty has always been greatly coveted. It is, after all, what you are, not what you have control over—like the ability to become powerful, successful, or famous—that is important in this business. Plastic surgery has, to some degree, helped those in pursuit of a desired "look," but you can't be taller or narrower than what nature made you. So within these boundaries the criteria of beauty are laid out.

The modeling world today dictates the statuesque figure of a nearly six-foot-tall female, with delicate bones and weighing no more than 115 pounds. That narrows the field immensely for those looking for a high-fashion modeling career. But many others have made successful modeling careers using only their beautiful faces or their perfectly proportioned figures.

CHAPTER 1

WHO ARE THE PROFESSIONAL MODELS?

Recently modeling has been singled out as a get-rich-quick profession. Since the main push worldwide is to amass personal monies, modeling has taken on a whole new reverence. International arenas are encompassing artists' models, runway models, photographic models, promotional models, television and video models, and showroom models. The entire gamut covers every age and every ethnic group. Basically, anyone is a potential model. Artists and photographers enlist a wide range of models in all sizes and shapes. And if you are truly determined to be a professional model, you probably will find some work in one capacity or another. Commercial artists work with the tiniest babies to the most aged grandparents, with the thinnest to the most corpulent bodies, and with the entire spectrum of ethnic backgrounds.

ARTISTS' MODELS

Sitting for an artist entails being a figure or a face that inspires that artist's creativity. What appeals to the artist's

1

taste or is needed to depict a certain idea will dictate what is required in the live model. Every body type and age group is included as the artist seeks inspiration.

Artists' models often start working in local art schools or for private painters, sculptors, or photographers as children. Sometimes it is the parent's wish that the child start working to make an income that will be used later for a specific reason, like education. At other times, the youngster is the one desirous of an early career. Working for an artist gives valuable training in discipline while teaching the model a bit about color, line, and style, if they are at all observant. The work entails holding a given pose for approximately five minutes, and then, after a short break, the pose is resumed. This can be very tedious to most individuals, and it is a very good test of potential patience for a future in modeling. If you are bored beyond belief, you'll not only have a tough time as a model regardless of the earnings, but you will not be a good model to the artist.

In addition, you will have to be available until the artistic rendering is completed, and that could be as short as a few hours or as long as a few months. Your patience and professionalism are critical, as many artists have that infamous artistic temperament. If you want the job, you'll have to be the one to comply, as most artists have very powerful personalities and strong convictions as to how their art will progress.

Art schools currently hire few, if any, child models, as they often have little discipline. However, you could find individual work or employment in some art schools for child students.

Most artists' models are between seventeen and seventy-five years of age. It is demanding work, but many choose to be associated with a talented artist as they enjoy the pleasure of feeling connected with the creation itself. Work can be found where artists gather, such as art schools, private galleries and studios, and classes held in art museums. You must contact these directly and follow their directions as far as getting an interview or an actual try out in front of a group of art students. There is also work to be found at college and university art and photographic classes. One job always leads to the next, so if you are mainly interested in remuneration from the modeling work, a little ingenuity goes a long way. The fashion institutes hire many models, and here is where the need becomes more specific. A female model must have the current fashion figure as well as poise and perhaps a bit of individual character. Often she must supply her own fashion wardrobe used in the model-sketching classes. Illustration classes also demand the model use her own wardrobe.

The pay scale in the New York area is around $10 an hour at the lowest level for the art schools and around $20 an hour for illustration classes. Different types of schools and individual artists pay varied scales as well. You will have to decide what you need and can afford to live on.

ILLUSTRATORS' MODELS

Illustrators are a special kind of artist used often in the fashion field to depict a more aesthetic face and figure than nature ever intended. For example, in our perversity, we like to see women who have no hips and look unnaturally thin. Somehow we think that clothing looks better on a creature unlike 99 percent of us because we are so unattractive. Well, this is where the illustrator comes in. He or she can and does make a drawing of someone taller than a tree and skinnier than a strand of angel hair pasta. Isn't it amazing to see the human model who sat for this rendering become stretched out like the reflection in a fun house mirror? There is a long-established department store in New York City that has employed fashion illustrators for more than two decades for all of its advertisements. You don't have to look at the store's name to identify it as its style of illustration has become its trademark—a form of advertising in itself.

As a model to a fashion illustrator, you will be paid very well. Some illustrators pay in the hundreds, while famous ones pay models thousands of dollars for a layout. If a celebrity model is used, her enormous pay scale would be met here as well. Some illustrators work from a photograph of the model, while others like to use the live model to view the different angles and present several renditions to the client. It is often believed to be quite prestigious to work with the world's top fashion illustrators as they are recognized artists and their work is very respected.

PROMOTIONAL MODELS

As you wend your way through hundreds of these live models who are selling everything from cosmetics to cars, you will be aware of one of the fastest-growing areas in the modeling world. The huge makeup companies were the first to see the potential for larger sales by having the model wear the products and also personally hawk the items. The department stores in New York City alone engage hundreds of these promo models every day. Most of them are not subtle in their approach. With atomizer in hand and free gift-with-purchase enticements, you are inundated with hordes of these models. So much selling has come to be done in this manner that the ranks now entail live models as well as promotional personnel. But the model is expected to be more the image or illusion that the company is trying to establish with the use of its product.

Sporty men, too, are seen in the employ of the clothing/ perfume makers for men. They wear some costume to link them to the product's theme and try to catch your attention with their attire and giveaways. The employment level here is still very much on the rise. Even the most humble of the clothing manufacturers now are promoting perfumes, where the big money really is to be made.

Annual promotional shows like the ones held at the Jacob Javit's Center in New York City also hire live models. These shows are seasonal and pay better than most other promotional modeling due to the very short period of work. As you can see, some verbal skill is required here. You may do as little as answer questions about a yacht that you are baby-sitting, or you may need to know every minute detail about a canned speech. Whatever the client needs, you'll have to be flexible enough to provide. It is not unusual now to be on some sort of commission as well as a salary if you are a promotional model. In general, this type of model is hired as new products need to be presented to the public—by week or month. A ballpark figure is around twenty dollars to several hundred dollars an hour for a very chic product promoted by an up-and-coming model. Benefits could ensue if you became the prime spokesperson/model for a specific product. You could find yourself with many big perks and great connections vis-à-vis the lowly promo job. So don't pass it by even if your heart is set on the more glamorous modeling areas. They could still come about while you're earning your way doing product presentations.

To land a promotional modeling job, contact companies and department stores that you'd like to work for. They will guide you in the right direction.

GARMENT OR FIT MODELS

The area around Seventh Avenue between the high twenties and the low forties in New York City is known as the garment district. It is within this section that nearly all the high-priced clothing made in the United States will be produced. The names that you recognize as "designer" manufacturers will be found here. It is very common for a pattern maker to select one girl for that house's size for its sample. The sample size varies with the desires of the American woman to shrink mentally while remaining the same size physically. This results in the strange phenomenon of sizes that zoom up in girth though the actual number remains the same. Men's clothing is not prone to this problem.

The fit model is usually about five feet nine inches tall and weighs about 118 pounds, ideally. This allows for a large variety in length of the torso and dimension of rib cage, bust, and hip. If you are seeking work as a fit model, look in the employment section of local newspapers.

Garment district establishments manufacture every kind of clothing imaginable from infant clothing to sportswear. They advertise seasonally and are usually looking for young female models as women are the greatest consumers of clothing in the country. Everything is modeled, from under-garments to evening gowns, so there are plenty of job opportunities.

This is not glamorous work as the employers are often brusque or shockingly demanding. If you are well man-nered, it might be a rude shock to you to work here, but it can be an experience that will help you assess your depth of desire to seek a modeling career. It is steady, pays the rent, and the good part is that if you can stand the pressure here, you can stand it anywhere. Jobs are generally by the week and pay approximately $100 to $150 per hour.

Seventh Avenue modeling is most beneficial if you can get work where you respect the designer and want to learn the ropes. Some girls are clever enough to make the leap from showroom to runway at the time of the seasonal presentations. It's rare but not impossible.

PHOTOGRAPHERS' MODELS

Here is the most desirous job in the industry. The women who have reached the pinnacle of modeling are all in this category. These are the now fresh-faced preteens who are astounding themselves with their quarter-million-dollar-a-year salaries. They arrive in the largest cities in droves with fame and fortune on their minds. The competition has never been more fierce, nor the ladder more slippery. Modeling has become the new road to riches for the eagerly independent, young neophyte.

A potential career in modeling has become so alluring to youngsters and their parents alike that we are now experiencing a frenzy to reach that goal. Modeling conventions have popped up all over the country and Canada; their fees, which are often in the thousands, make these popular events a gold mine for promoters. Young men and women believe that if they pay their way in they will be discovered. Unfortunately, only a handful out of a thousand will even get a callback, let alone a contract. A contract with any agent does not even guarantee you a modeling career! Open call by the agents themselves show that one in a thousand is given a callback.

Some wanna-bes have been persistent enough to go to one agent after another if rejected, and that would seem sensible enough. It would appear that with the given statistics, it might be best to just go to every open call that you can and leave your face-and-figure shot. Even young men are now in here battling their way to the agencies. It is obvious that the expectation, or even just the hope of success, will float the youngster. Great sums of money have been made by the superdivas—six and a half million to one celebrity for her year's efforts. But it is very unlikely that you're going to get the gold at the end of the great runway. So do try to be realistic. Years ago there simply was no celebrity associated with the modeling world, and thus there was less crazed competition even for the smallest job.

The photographic model includes everyone from the baby in diapers to the high-fashion mannequin in the international marketplace. Catalog work is still among the most common bread-and-butter work for all ages, sexes, and ethnic groups. There is a huge boom in the mail order catalog business, and it has and continues to guarantee many jobs for models. The pay starts at around $150 per hour and goes up, depending on your fees commanded by the agency.

"Real" people are used in many catalogs now as opposed to a few years back, when, for example, a totally unbelievable scene showed a buxom blond hand-mowing the lawn.

There are also "part" models who are not a totally salable package. They may have perfect teeth for a toothpaste commercial, an elegant and long leg for a stocking ad, or luxuriant hair for a shampoo clip. You can see how many niches there are in the photographic area of modeling. All of them pay exceedingly well, and many give you an introduction to the next job.

Photographic work is available in the smallest town to the most sophisticated city. There is a recent upswing of work in Texas and Canada in particular, as they enter the fashion world more fully. The number of modeling agencies in these two areas has tripled in the last ten years.

RUNWAY MODELS AND FASHION-SHOW WORK

In the past few years, there has been an unbelievable phenomenon on the fashion runway. It has become a social event of the highest order. The queens of the runway shows include about a dozen high-fashion divas who work every big name designer's presentation in Paris and Italy. The United States does not have the old-name fashion houses at this level, and haute couture is the real showstopper of the fashion world. When these shows are given, they are such social happenings that hotels are booked a year in advance. It is no wonder that the supermodels can command such high salaries when the shows that they work draw masses of millionaires just dying to buy these garments before someone else does. It's a little like Evita. She knew enough to want the very best. And when the gowns are selling for $350,000 each, you can understand the model who says that she is what made the gown look so desirable and, thus, demands her share, too.

One fashion supermodel also received the salary of $60,000 for seventy-two hours of work on the runway. The women need tremendous stamina, even though they look like they would blow over in a wind. They appear in endless shows during a few insanely hectic weeks.

The haute couture clothing is the really fabulous costume of which dreams are made. There is no limit to cost of fabric, dramatic presentation, or talent. The runway at this level has replicated show business wherein the "actresses" need do nothing but walk and turn, and rarely smile. Experience does count for something here, as you see the same models over and over, year after year. Partially because the recognizable model becomes like the recognized designers she represents does all this add up to a form of social status.

The public has always wanted to emulate the rich and the famous, and fashion makes them feel that this is attainable by copying these runway clothes. The really great costumes that ensure the designer's creative recognition are rarely worn by anyone except the models, but the street gear is simply not as fantastic, stunning, or, frankly, as much fun to wear. It is not by accident that the couture designer presents the pièce de résistance in the form of a breathtaking, celestial wedding gown as the last statement in his or her collection. It is what fashion and modeling is all about, illusion at its most mystical level.

The fashion model who is invited to do the runway is certainly already a supermodel or nearing that status. These shows are patronized by not only those who can afford to buy the creations (though they are the most necessary) but by the fashion industry, its editors, its manufacturers, and its thousands of links in the chain: hair stylists, accessory makers, makeup artists, and armies of others who are attached to this area of chic.

The runway model usually is not a young teenage girl, but a late teens to late twenties woman with some serious experience. The casual strut dominating the runway comes from years of working what is familiarly referred to as the *catwalk.* The near-bored-to-death glances from the models probably are more real than theatrical, but it's all part of the portrayal of the semijaded attitude so popular in status culture.

Different parts of the world offer different levels of runway work. You will be able to find these jobs in areas as small as your local mall, in small cities at business lunches, for charities on hotel stages, in Seventh Avenue houses, and worldwide wherever fashion exists.

There are also men models on the runways, though rarely is there anywhere near the same hoopla for them. They are, however, beginning to be seen annually on the runways of Paris, Milan, and New York in innovative clothing at big designer's shows. There are simply no comparisons between the celebrity models who are all women and any of the men models. The public can name many of these lady divas, but the male model neither commands the runway nor the gigantic celebrity and its accompanying salaries. Image leads to income, and this is very much a female-beauty dominated world. According to one modeling association, the women model's income outranks the men's by fifty to one hundred times per annum!

One of the biggest modeling agencies in the world is said to represent nearly four times as many women as men. Products and fashion are more often purchased by or for women than men, so the models for these products are the likely persons to be seen with them. The fashion world since Louis XVI has been pretty much one of interest to the female, though that is changing somewhat with the attempts to clothe successful men in something other than blue pin-striped suits.

The runway model is the greatest beauty that the industry can find. These women are tall, leggy, lean, pretty, and have a bit of a bosom. The male runway model must be slender, have nicely developed chest muscles, and be that near classic size 40. He must exude a sexy quality, whatever that is defined as at the moment. Currently it is the unshaven, or clean-cut, or movie star look-alike look. Statistics show that American men purchase what they need and that fashion per se is only considered by one-fourth of them. With those numbers is it any wonder that men's fashions are still primarily dress suits and casual attire like jeans? There simply aren't as many opportunities for the male model as there are for the females.

MALE MODELS

The male model is still climbing the ladder and making inroads into the female-dominated trade. There is more work now than ever for male models. With the advent of fashion shows and runway work, men are starting to be more visible, and they are beginning to want the big salaries that women models have enjoyed for many years.

The male market appeals to fashion-conscious men, and as such it must be innovative. Recently a new style of men's suit was introduced. Whether it catches on in the conservative world of men's classic needs will remain to be seen. It would appear that the exact proportion of men interested in the fashion world of clothing at the buyer's level equals the number of models hired. The current proportion is 25 percent of men to women models and that same number at the polls are current fashion trend buyers!

While the female model is exaggerated in height, weight, and exotic look, the male model is usually about six feet tall and weighs around 170 pounds. He and the size 40 suit seem eternal. The truth is that no matter how much the retail business and the designers for men would like to entice a new buying market, it's very small in catching on. Men purchase the uniform requested by their place of work and some casual clothing for days off, but unless they need specialized clothing for, say, horseback riding or soccer, they are very unlikely to buy clothing. Just getting a tuxedo for a formal occasion can cause near apoplexy in most men!

If you are interested in working as a male model, I would offer you the same advice as I do for women. Avoid putting any money up front. Go directly to the largest city within your budget and have an interview at several agencies that you already have contacted. Open calls are great, too; only the competition scares some potential models off. There are scores of model competitors out there anyway, so the sooner you learn to deal with it all, the better for you.

You must have a look that the agent believes he or she can sell. Most larger agencies have their own men's models division, and if you just peruse the men's fashion magazines, you will quickly assess the looks currently in vogue. The want ads in large city newspapers as well as the Seventh Avenue papers to the trade will advertise for male models and will have job listings for fit models and some show and runway work. An agent is surely the best avenue to work in all the areas: catalog, photograph, print, TV, video, and even work for illustrators.

TELEVISION MODELS

Anywhere that you find the astronomical salaries paid for commercials, you'll find actors and models battling it out. If the role does not call for speaking on the air, a model is usually acceptable, and a lot less expensive, to the client. Once an actor with a union affiliation is used, you are usually talking about a $20,000 payment. Last year alone, $1.4 billion were earned by Screen Actors' Guild (SAG) holding contracts. It is no mystery why any model would love to have one of these union cards. Anyone could be a television model from the baby just able to sit to the aged who could do ads for elderly products. Many famous people like sports figures and movie stars also do TV commercials, so the competition is the most frenzied here. Jobs are to be found in any trade paper or periodical, at modeling agencies, or through personal agents.

Sometimes it is simply the ability to do something that few people are capable of or afraid of trying that will land the job. For a while there was a call for bungee jumpers, rock climbers, and hang gliders. As these extreme sports gain in popularity, so will the jobs in commercials for these unique individuals. A voice-over is used in nearly all of these commercials, and the model is merely seen, not heard.

The television commercial is so widely known for making big money that many liken it to winning the lottery. Television casting directors are inundated with thousands of applicants for every commercial. Auditions weed out the masses, and if you are lucky enough to get a callback, it's nearly a miracle. But someone will be chosen, and it could be you. There are ways to improve these odds, and the first step nowadays is to go to acting classes geared toward commercials and learn how to present yourself, as well as make it through the cattle-call auditions that can be devastating.

There are tricks to every trade, and modeling for TV commercials is no different. One believable bottle-blond has done nothing but shampoo commercials for years, and she is still typecast. It often happens that you'll click in a particular area and the money is so stupendous, that you can live on one or two commercials' income for a year. The acting classes that I mentioned above are for children as well as adults and are given in most big cities. There are many supermodels doing TV commercials for huge sums of money as well as little cherubs spitting out baby food for tidy double-digit thousands of dollars. Being a TV model could bring you that union card and the doubled salary for simply being seen and not heard.

VIDEO MODELS

There are millions of videos made annually, and many of them entail professional modeling. You can see dozens of video machines rolling in boutiques and department stores. The demonstrations could be anything from blowing up a mattress to cooking with innovative pots and pans.

Models are often employed to discuss deployment of safety gear for airplanes, describe how to sell a particular product to a sales staff, and even do visual inventories like jewelry in a boutique. The possibilities are endless, and though pretty faces and hands are usually enough of a pre-requisite to endorse these products, sometimes type characters are employed as well. Many men's products, such as men's perfumes, luggage, and clothing, are sold using male models. Although the runway shows that are presented live in Italy, Paris, and the United States are videotaped and shown to the masses, models are paid once and there are no residuals like in TV.

Children demonstrating toys, high fashion models wearing full makeup for the client's company, and all the articles that you have ever seen or heard of could potentially be on video. The video camera is so popular now that we see television shows based solely on its use.

Depending on what the client has in mind, the model may or may not have to speak. Acting always looks easy to those who have never tried it as they assume models are simply being themselves. In truth, most individuals will overact in this situation. A camera that captures you in an instant shot will surely give away all your insecure motions in a video. Just watch the nervous eye motion or twitching hands of a person being videotaped. Calmness must be acquired. It is a dead giveaway that you don't exude confidence in yourself or the product if your exclamations are punctuated with your hands moving faster than your mouth!

Video could work tremendously to your advantage as your resume or as an example of your look as a model. Videos taken of you doing the unique things that you are qualified to incorporate into your modeling work could also be door openers. Agents and casting directors are bored to tears with the same old presentations, so that little extra eye-catching possible from a video may land you the job, and that's what this is all about—selling yourself first to the agent, then to the client.

The pay scale for video work depends solely on how big the client is and what he or she intends to do with the tape. It could mean as little as a few hundred dollars to double-digits in the thousands.

CHAPTER 2

ATTRIBUTES NEEDED FOR MODELING

LOOKS AND ATTITUDE

Modeling agencies employ hundreds of "workhorse" models and a handful of supermodels. The masses of the former group go on the thousands of interviews set up by their agencies in the hope of being the right stuff. You must sell yourself as the best model for the money and image to be made. The agency merely makes the contact and you are the sale clincher. Here is where personality and character count. It has become fashionable to depict a sullen, bored, or even a cynical expression in fashion shoots, but the attitude I am discussing here is one of professionalism only.

If you don't appear hungry for the work and thus available for every go-see, your agency will simply not try to get work for you. If you are easily discouraged by rejection, this is not a potential career. An optimistic attitude is paramount, and even if you've struck out for the last dozen go-sees, you'll have to appear fresh and ready to go every time you're interviewed by a client,

Desire to reach a certain goal is the only driver that you will have. The agent is merely there to bridge the gap between you and the patron at a set price to you. How fast you reach your destination in modeling is in your hands only.

Keep your eye on your goal. If you are rejected on a go-see, don't take it personally. If you never made the effort to get there, that's a different story. Your agency will keep trying for your probationary period just as long as you do. Even the most gorgeous person alive doesn't become a model instantly. Hard work derived from your innermost desire to be a model is the only way to make it.

A professional attitude toward yourself and your work is the next criterion. There are few other professions where you are so completely representing the marketable product (in this case *you*) in total. The client, your agency, the photographers, and even the stylists *will* be looking and remembering. You need to be remembered for that next job and future jobs. It is of paramount importance that you are remembered for being a pleasure to work with in every way. This means being physically appealing, neat, immaculately clean, clean shaven (women and men), and having impeccable hair and nails. Many jobs are lost by models who are simply careless about personal care. When a model is not absolutely fastidious about cleanliness, an employer or client probably will not call that person for a job ever again.

Clean and neat clothing from undergarments outward are a real boon. One male model states that (early in his career) he was made very aware that agents as well as clients were scrutinizing his garments as part of his total appearance. The call-backs that he has received have proven him to be right. Even if you don't have an extensive wardrobe, be certain that you appear in fresh-looking garments that are of as good quality as you can possibly afford.

With all the current advertising emphasis on designers' names, you will want to own clothing that is recognizable as chic to those whom you are trying to impress. It's not a must that you have any identifying labels. But you must demonstrate your fashion awareness by a generally "in" look or costume. Observe other models' get-ups as they dress for go-sees. There is such a wide variance in self-sell modes that once you are a little more sure of your placement in the modeling agency, you are a bit freer to set differing looks for different jobs. Models—known and not so well established—can be seen on their way to jobs in New York City in everything from really ratty jeans to exquisite suits with a full complement of accessories. Both ends of the fashion spectrum are worn by models. The correct timing is the all-important key to when it's right to wear what.

What is really unique to New York City is the personal mix of what amounts to fashion. Mink and blue jeans, evening gowns and vintage wraps, casual and formal wear in one costume are all part of the current fashion scene, so you are pretty much able to "do it yourself," as long as the final creation is within a certain arena. That arena changes rapidly, and the really avant garde always have the most fun with clothing. In fashion you can't be a follower, but if you get too far ahead of the pack, you're just that. Keep a keen eye on the current fashion trends, and *try* to dress as you will be expected to as a representative of a specific client of the fashion world.

PHYSICAL QUALIFICATIONS FOR HIGH FASHION

First on the list is *youth!* Many high fashion models as young as thirteen years of age are involved in career modeling. Their annual incomes rank among the highest salaries paid to any workers, including corporate executives, doctors, and attorneys. These very young girls are the beauties whose figures and faces are seen daily in publications and on television. All of them are between the ages of perhaps eleven to twenty-three. The really great high fashion model can stretch her career into her middle to late twenties, if she is very lucky. That is truly an unusual phenomenon, though, so the earlier you start, the better your chances are at making a career in this field.

The second qualification is that your height must be somewhere between five feet ten inches and six feet four. A really stunning beauty at five feet eight and a half inches could get by. The idea here is proportionate height with very slender limbs. So, if you are extremely fine boned though shorter, you might still have a chance at high fashion work.

Weight is critical. You cannot weigh more than 115 pounds, and that would be on the tallest frame. Most of the models weigh around 110 to 115. Your weight has to stay consistent. This is accomplished by sticking to a highly restricted diet and by exercising.

The weight must be distributed proportionately over your frame. You must not have any bulges or even any visible bumps. Long and slender is the guide. Arms, legs, torso, and neck should be as lean as the proverbial race horse. The bust is usually not larger than a B cup, but you could look into lingerie work if you are larger. Long, lanky, and nicely shaped legs are critical. Much of fashion depends on the height of the model and how the garment looks on the over-tall frame. The desired spot to carry the extra height is in the leg, not the torso or neck.

Another important characteristic is that you must have a very photogenic face. This usually means straight features that are rather small. If you want to do runway work exclusively, you need not worry about being photogenic, but most models in the high fashion category combine all the areas possible to round out their careers, as well as their incomes. If you have some snapshots that look pretty bad, don't assume that you do not photograph well. It may be that all you need is a good professional photographer who will take the time to work with you. Few models photograph the way they really look. The camera can lie, and it's not a sure bet in which way! Sometimes an incredible beauty looks almost ugly and vice versa.

Your face can make a tremendous difference not only in your potential income but in your total life as a model. The right combination of attractive eyes, alignment of nose, and alluring mouth could be the difference between an average model and a million dollar one.

Look in the mirror and honestly assess what you see. Makeup does help tremendously, but the bottom line basics are the aforementioned, plus no visible marks. If you have any scars, beauty marks, heavy freckles, or real variance in structure, they could count against you. Some freckles are considered to be very much in vogue, particularly in cases where the model is endowed with gorgeous red hair and golden or blue to green eyes.

Trying to change your physical attributes through plastic surgery is possible but advisable only if you are genuinely unhappy with part of your face—perhaps a small scar or mark. Modeling can be extremely fickle. What is "in" today could be as unpopular next month as the flu. Many times a model has been advised to have rhinoplasty only to have a worse nose afterward or to discover that the original is now what is in style. Noses with bumps in the bridge, bushy eyebrows, slightly crooked smiles, irregular jaw lines, and ill-matched eyes are just a few of the trendy flaws that come and go in fashion work. Don't outguess the agents; what you consider an imperfection, they may be able to turn into a desirable characteristic.

Hair, teeth, and skin must be healthy, attractive, and vibrant. An all-around complement of appealing good looks is critical.

Some high fashion designers seek out a certain "look" for their collections, a look that is instantly recognizable for their particular lines or collections. If you look at the fashion spreads, you will be able to see at a glance what style is developed by each designer. Some are enchanted with the classic beauty, with fair hair and skin, light eyes, small tipped-up nose, and a generally English countryside appearance. Other designers prefer sultry brunettes to carry off the look of their collections. It is the complete impression of the coloring and facial expression of the high fashion model that is sought after for much live and photographic work.

Different modeling agencies actually specialize in these various looks, and the largest agencies are able to supply everything from cute to sultry-looking models, depending on the client's needs. Some newer models try to develop a single look that they will be known for. Others are as wide-ranging in their look as a chameleon; you would really not believe that it could be the same person from page to page in a layout. Clever makeup, hair styles, and clothing can and do create totally different presentations to the public's eye.

The different looks that you will be required to create are affected by not only the costume, makeup, and scenery, but by a mood you communicate through facial and body expressions. The most clever models are good at mime; they can represent an action, character, mood, or feeling by imitation. Some articles of clothing lend themselves to a certain feeling on the part of the model. Imagination is critical, as there are often situations in which you are handed an item and are expected to wing it.

Movement is an asset for the would-be model, as there isn't an easy way to learn the actions needed by the fashion world without a little innate grace and skillful emulation. Opinions differ as to the easiest way to acquire the necessary agility. Rhythm does not come easily to everyone, so the earlier that you become engaged in some kind of dance, sports, or music, the easier the art of moving well and with confidence will develop. If you have poise and self-assurance, moving like a high fashion model will be simple enough to learn. But if you have to start from the very beginning even to have ease of movement, you could be in trouble. Even as a young adult, poor carriage and stilted motions are a giveaway that you are really ill at ease, and this is a profession in which your basic job is to convey absolute self-confidence.

To have the winning combination of desire, great looks, height, slenderness, poise, facial beauty, proportionate figure, and youth is to be in possession of the right physical characteristics for a high fashion model. There are, of course, emotional and professional characteristics required as well. These are discussed elsewhere in this book.

QUALIFICATIONS FOR ALL MODELS

Physical good health is paramount for modeling. The stress can be intense, the hours brutal, the positions difficult, the travel wearing, and the weather trying for outdoor work. If you don't feel in top-notch shape, you're simply not going to last as long as you're required to, and exhaustion will cost everyone from your agency to the client.

Discipline is rigid for every model, children included. You must keep a consistent weight, build, and all-around "look." Your diet and exercise regimen must be strictly followed, and eight hours of sleep is critical for you to look and perform well.

Patience is a virtue you will need every time you have an interview, a go-see, or a session. Sometimes there are delays and hitches that make you want to scream. Keep calm. Hysterics will make you an instantly unpopular model, and the others who can hold up under pressure will be the ones asked for return engagements. There is nothing worse than helping to make a bad situation a disaster, so try to remain cool while others lose their tempers. You'll be remembered and rewarded.

Enthusiasm makes the really great models. Sprightly young models are the mainstay of the business. They promote everything from foods to bobby pins with an effervescent quality that often appears to be genuine. It has been said by agents that the person with the greatest charm, sparkle, and passion can compete successfully with the greater natural beauty who lacks fire.

You must be able to take rejection as a daily diet without getting depressed. Every time you are sent on a go-see, the chances are that you only "may" get that job. Many people compete for each job. You must keep a permanently optimistic view toward your career and yourself. This is the hardest part for many models, because rejection does make you feel discouraged. You have to keep trying and trying and trying. That seventh or eighth go-see just may be the plum that you've prayed for.

You need an endless ability to take criticism and work with it. You may be asked or even rudely told to do something like hold a very difficult pose. For all of your serious endeavors, it may not work. After agonizing for some time, the tempers begin to flare. You, as the model, are the target, and you simply have to keep trying to get it right. Criticizing is the only way the photographer is able to elicit the best shots, and if you're not an instantaneous "natural" (and about one in a million is "at home" in front of camera, photographer, and stylists all demanding at once), then you have to give a thousand percent every time you are asked to do a job. The cooperation of everyone is really visible in the final product.

You will be well-advised to have a sense of humor. Things can and do go wrong. A sense of humor can relieve the tension so that progress can be resumed.

You must keep yourself organized. This means being fully prepared for every job promptly, enthusiastically, and professionally. You can *never* be late to a go-see or an actual job! That is an unforgivable transgression. It keeps an entire group of people (who are getting paid) waiting, and you may never see another job through your agency again. Everyone has a schedule to meet, and your major responsibility is to get there on time! Excuses are unacceptable in this trade. If you are genuinely ill or there is a real crisis, you are expected to call your agency at the earliest moment so that the fewest people will be inconvenienced by the change in schedule.

You will be expected to be congenial and yet not socialize. Everyone there is ready to work, and it is very difficult for some to realize that this is an atmosphere of serious and hard endeavor. You must not get carried away with the idea of being a star, but realize that this is primarily work and that if you let yourself slip into an unhealthy frame of mind, it could have some serious repercussions. One very successful, internationally known model says that it is quite common for new men and women to blow their whole potential career with their attitudes of superiority and subsequent lack of professionalism. They get caught up in the myth that models are glamorous and terrific, and they forget how replaceable they are. Many other models are waiting in the wings.

You must realize at this juncture that you will not be able to have a full social life. When all of your friends are ready to start the night's activities, you will be bowing out for an early night's sleep. When you are expected to look sensational at six in the morning, that means showing up looking rested and fresh, not haggard and with bags under your eyes. The only models who can get by with a normal social calendar are the television subjects for cold remedy and sleeping tablet commercials. Modeling is a difficult and highly disciplined way of life. Before choosing it, you should weigh the sacrifices against the rewards.

QUALIFICATIONS FOR MALE MODELS

Male modeling has come into its own and can now be considered a true career area for men. A few years ago, the major work for the male model was work as a backup to the high fashion model or catalog work. The field has expanded so much that most modeling agencies have opened sections for the men only. The criterion used to be the size 40 regular suit. Now there is a little variation, though not too much in either direction. The main thing that the agencies are looking for in the male model is a really appealing face and slender body. The current look is from clean-cut collegiate, to swarthy unshaven ruggedness.

The photogenic requirement is critical here, as that is the basic bread-and-butter area for men. Runway modeling is a new field for men, and though you might not need to be photogenic for that specific job, most runway work using male models is being videotaped. There is so little work for the male model that does not involve photography that he should not seriously consider a career in the field unless the camera is kind to him.

Agencies are looking for men between six feet and six feet two inches tall who lend themselves to the "look" that the agencies represent. A pseudorugged look is currently in vogue.

If you have the basic criteria, send a few snapshots to a local agency or even the largest agencies. If they think you have the potential, they'll advise you. Then if you are in the area, you'll want to set up an interview to confirm that you have what the agent needs. The agency will then set about helping you to acquire really good photographs (testing), so that your pictures will fit the requirements. They will guide you and turn you into a polished model with the look that will be beneficial to both them and you.

The more unique facial features are most in demand. Look through men's fashion magazines and keep an eye on newspaper photographs of the current popular male models to get an idea of the needed features, haircuts, bone structures, and coloring.

Pretty teeth, sparkling or sensual eyes, and a fairly straight nose are required. Smaller features are the most fashionable looking. That lovely combination of perfect proportion in facial features and slender, tall body are the winning criteria for the male model.

Black and exotic male models are needed in all of the various areas of modeling. The ages of male models are more widespread than those of the females. A man in the field could last from his teens through his forties, as long as he maintains his good looks and his slender frame.

Catalogs have been known to show a male model over a span of twenty years! One male model who is still working and is in his fifties looks as if he is in his mid-thirties. His self-discipline has been extraordinarily consistent, and it has paid off. He has been a professional male model for over thirty years and has made a very nice living with his chosen career.

QUALIFICATIONS FOR CHILD MODELS

Children are used in modeling for catalogs, television, and print ads. Child models are required to be very well behaved and cooperative. Although you cannot expect adult behavior, absolute compliance is critical since they are working and are being paid for such. Child models must be unique, charming, appealing, cute, or pretty. They must be a perfect size. They must be photogenic, and they must want to work. It's not enough that they have all of the potential, unless they themselves desire to model.

The pay scale is enough to make any parent consider the prospects, but the child is the one who will be doing the sitting, so make sure that he or she really wants to work. If you have a child who you think might make a good model, send snapshots to an agency in your area, and they will get back to you if they are interested. Be sure to include a letter telling the child's statistics: clothing and shoe sizes, age, hair and eye coloring (if shots are black-and-white), height, and weight.

A Word of Caution to Parents

If you are considering a modeling career for your child, be sure to write to your local labor department for any work permits required by your particular state. There are several other permits required by various groups to protect the child, and your agency will advise you of these.

If you or your child is considering a television commercial as a source of income, check with the various unions such as SAG (Screen Actors' Guild) and AFTRA (American Federation of Television and Radio Artists). You are only permitted to do your first commercial without membership in these unions.

QUALIFICATIONS FOR TELEVISION MODELS

Anyone *could* be a television model. That covers the entire gamut of physical characteristics from babies to grandmothers. The most often-used models are young, pretty women who promote products. Aside from the high fashion model, whose criteria we discussed earlier, these women could be anywhere from petite to amazon in structure, and the men could have any look from the innocent little boy to the grumpy insomniac. The variations are endless.

There are two distinct parts of television modeling. You must be extroverted, determined, and self-assured to do the modeling, but you must also be capable of speaking for the medium if you're going to be doing the talking as well. You'll want to take lessons if you can't make the second half of the criteria, as the models who talk are the ones who get paid doubly. There is no such thing as being a wrong type for TV work; it's merely a matter of waiting until the demand for your look comes along. There are people who are very talented and appear time and again in commercials. They develop different characters for every ad. These models are often professional actors who have the advantage of not only having a look but also a particular chameleon ability. If you are seriously considering TV work, try to do a little acting, and then contact a local agency to see what kind of head shot they require; include it with your resume at your interview.

CHAPTER 3

BREAKING INTO MODELING

Many models are fortunate in having a mother or a friend who has had experience in the modeling world and can offer personal advice. Inside information certainly smooths the way in a profession that can be potentially unpleasant or even risky. Youth and ambition are a combination that could make you easy prey if you are not aware of very unscrupulous persons who could be waiting to take advantage of you. This profession is particularly rife with pitfalls, and you will need someone to look out for you, especially in a large fast city. Where beautiful and very young girls are treated as commodities, it is often difficult to keep the path clear of hazards.

With this in mind, look for the modeling agency with the most pristine reputation for safeguarding its models. The agency that takes precautions and carefully selects its clients will be in business with a secure future. You need only look at the Yellow Pages to see how quickly an agency can fail. Few modeling agencies last more than a very few seasons. A handful of seasoned modeling agencies continue to exist after five years' time.

ARE YOU MODEL MATERIAL?

If you live in an area far from major cities, you will have to rely on your own hunches and trying to establish yourself as being attractive in the local public eye. It is difficult without having the advantage of the professional's experience to judge, but you generally know if you might have the potential. That is the starting point.

If you've already been noticed by local photographers or been considered good-looking by others all your life, you are probably at least attractive. The only way to know what that might mean for you as a model is to proceed in the general direction of public affirmation of your physical attributes. Popularity must not be confused with possible modeling qualifications.

After reading Chapter 1 of this book, you should have a better idea where you fit in. The dictates are pretty clear-cut, so don't expect an agency to make exceptions. If your reflection shows you a short, rounded figure with hips and sloping shoulders, don't torture yourself by trying to be what you're not. There are millions of job opportunities in the world. If your heart's desire is to be in the modeling world, maybe you could be happy in a model-associated field. Or maybe you would be satisfied as a specialty model who has some perfect parts like hands, face, or smile. It is obviously more difficult to test the waters for your potential ability in rural areas. Your best bet might be to have some good photographs made of your hands or some good head shots and send them with a covering letter and a resume to an agency. If they are interested, they will make an appointment with you. Many modeling schools in smaller city areas are good sources of contact. When you take classes with them, it often entitles you to do regional modeling work.

You need lots of exposure to get a good handle on public response to your ability to model. The tinier the geographical area, the harder it will be to gain this kind of exposure, but there are endless ways to expand this limitation. After you have contacted the modeling schools, make an effort to write or talk to all the agencies in nearby cities. From there, you may want to enter all the local beauty contests and visit all the department stores and malls, leaving your name and photo (with your statistics and phone number). You may be surprised at the amount of work that can come your way in this manner. If a model is needed for a promotion, and you were clever enough to have left all the needed information, you will probably be the first chosen. It's happened more often than one would suppose that a "break" was prepared ahead of time by an aspirant, and luck did the rest. There is just too much competition for these jobs for you to be able to sit back and wait for them to come to you.

Suppose you are doing all right in a medium-sized city as a model. You may be perfectly happy there, and though the money is not earthshaking, you could make a decent living ($20,000 to $30,000) keeping quite busy with runway work, promotional work, photographic work, and whatever local television work you could pick up. You are in demand and available full-time. If you are totally dependent upon your modeling wages, make certain to have a nest egg to tide you over, as modeling is often affected by fickle trends.

As a high fashion model hopeful, you will have to make your way to New York City, Los Angeles, or Chicago. Two smaller cities with moderate amounts of work to offer would be Atlanta and Cleveland in the east, and San Francisco and Dallas in the west. You may want to give these latter cities a try before you feel confident enough to approach the capitals of modeling.

Any positive experience under your belt will be an added plus in your climb up the ladder in a modeling career.

THE BEAUTY CONTEST

Thousands of aspiring young women have entered local beauty pageants in the hope of being discovered as models, starlets, and eventual celebrities. These contests are always open to pretty or talented girls. Some even include women who have grown children! There is so much chance for media coverage in these contests that even if you are not any more than a local winner, you could get quite a bit of mileage out of the publicity. There are also the added incentives of prizes and possible scholarships and contracts. It can be a surprisingly good stepping-stone.

Agents and their assistants have a keen eye focused on the many contests that occur annually. Many an ignored contestant has become a top model, partly because beauty pageants are geared toward a much meatier body than fashion modeling and partly because many beauty contestants photograph well but do not come across well in personal appearances (critical to the mass promotions on such contests). There is no longer a stigma on entering to win, and it is not unusual to see last year's Miss State XYZ be this year's representative of State ZYX, having established residency in the six months required to qualify. And amazingly, these women time and again walk off with the prizes the second, third, or even fourth time around. There is obviously something to be said for their methodical approaches.

Very few people would want to make a career of vying annually for places in beauty pageants, but as far as a lesson in persistence goes, it is similar to the attitude that you'll need to have for modeling. If you are convinced that you really want to get into modeling, there are hundreds of beauty contests available to you. Start by reading the magazines geared to the teenage market, and carefully select those contests that offer modeling jobs as prizes. There are many such contests, but the entry fees may be costly and the wardrobe another out-of-pocket expense. Some contests are so costly that sponsors are available, and you will have to investigate which ones will promote you the best toward your modeling goal.

A local pageant may give you the experience that will help you get to the top in a bigger one, or you may want to try for the nationals right away.

One major drawback in the two largest contests (Miss America and Miss Universe) is the age requirement for entering. If you are young and heart-set on a high fashion career, you may do better to give the smaller contests your attention, as they are geared to teenagers exclusively. Youth being the marketable item that it is, you may be wasting precious time by holding out for bigger stakes.

The most well-known beauty contests for teenagers are given in the following list. It is best for you to write directly to each for information regarding the time, place, entry fees, and rules. So study the regulations and be aware of what they can do to help your career get started.

Miss Teenage America
  Teen Magazine
  110 Fifth Avenue
  New York, NY 10011

America's Junior Miss Austin
  (Texas Junior Miss Pageant)
  (512) 454-5395

Miss Teenage California Pageant
  For official application call:
  (916) 684-4225

Miss Austin Scholarship Pageant
  5715 Burnet Road
  Austin, TX 78756

America's Junior Miss Pageant
  751 Government Street
  Mobile, AL 36602

Miss Black America Pageant
  (215) 844-8872

Miss California Pageant, Inc.
  P.O. Box 293
  San Diego, CA 92112

Ms. United States of America
  Pageant
  1075 Bellvue Way, NE
  Bellvue, WA 98004

Miss America Pageant
  Boardwalk Arcade Building
  Boardwalk and Tennessee
  Avenue
  Atlantic City, NJ 08401

Miss Ohio Pageant, Inc.
  P.O. Box 1818
  Mansfield, OH 44901

The aforementioned contests can give you great exposure and lots of press coverage. With all the photography and television, you will be able to get an idea of how you look on film. There are many local contests that lead up to the bigger ones, and every inch of the way could help your modeling career along. As long as you hold even the most insignificant title, people are curious to see what and who you are, so don't hesitate to push yourself forward for even the smallest contests. Modeling is nothing but competition at the bottom line, and every chance to compete should be welcomed.

The more experience the better. The competition must be overcome in such a way that you come out on top looking like you were just the best choice, not clawing tooth and nail to push yourself to the forefront. Everything has been tried, from researching the judges' backgrounds (to better prepare answers that would please their interests), to extensive plastic surgery (in the hope of being just what the judges are looking for). You'll do best by sticking with what you already have. Beauty contests are judged by human beings whose ideas of beauty are often very different. You could spend your entire life arranging yourself to suit someone else's likes or expectations.

Two other competitions in particular are conducted with a modeling contract offered as a prize. The most famous is Super Model of the World/Face of the 90's (in association with Ford Models, Inc.), and the other is *Teen's* Great Model Search.

Super Model of the World

The international search for Super Model of the World will take place every fall throughout the world. To enter, contact the Ford agency in New York City. Ask for the super model division. As the contest will differ slightly every year, the most up-to-date information will be available from Ford Models, Inc. Their address can be found under the listings of agencies and schools in the back of this book. You must be between fourteen and twenty-four to enter. They will want to know your name, address, telephone number, date of birth, measurements, height, and weight. You will also need to enclose two snapshots or larger photographs: one head shot, one body shot. They need not be professional shots, and either black and white or color ones are acceptable.

If you win the regional contest, you will continue to compete in the United States until one girl is selected who will enter the international contest as the United States representative. The final contest is held annually at a different exotic location.

The coveted prize is a modeling contract for $250,000 for a three-year period.

Teen's Great Model Search

Teen's Great Model Search has no physical stipulations as to height and weight. This competition requires head and full body shots and all statistics. Entrants must be from the United States or Canada, be between the ages of twelve and eighteen, and desire to become a model. For more information write to Great Model Search, *Teen Magazine,* 110 Fifth Avenue, 5th floor, New York, NY 10011.

HEADING FOR THE BIG AGENCIES

If you already live in or near New York City, Chicago, or Los Angeles, you may want to approach the top people in the field. The big agencies are naturally where the largest amounts of money can be made, and if you are truly qualified, why shouldn't you start at the highest salary that you can command?

Call and make an appointment with an interviewer. Some agencies prefer that you bring photographs so that the interviewer can see how photogenic you are. If you only have bad shots of yourself and you realize that they are awful, *don't take them* to an agent. The scrutinizing eye of the agent will be able to tell whether you should invest in *any* shots. They might not be interested at all, and then you would be wasting your money and time. On the other hand, if you have good photographs of your face and full body, you will certainly want to show them to the agent. The agent will be looking at how well your bone structure comes across in a photograph.

The interviewers' keen eye is really critical in delineation of potential models. Their experience in what to look for can save you many hours of indecision. If you are just what that particular agency needs, you may happily end your search. If not, you must make another and another appointment until you have exhausted all of the agencies, large and small, that you would consider working for.

Give yourself a fair chance to get into an agency. After several months and some polishing of your whole look, however, if you are still pounding the sidewalks, start to think of another profession. The experts really do know, and there's very little that can be done to change the current selling look.

BREAKING INTO TELEVISION MODELING

Many models are already working as photographic models when they make the first step into the television commercial. Such people are guided by their agents and are prepared for the audition so that they know what to expect. An audition of any kind can be a pretty awful experience, and it is particularly noted for its destruction of egos. Of course if you *do* land the part, you can feel really elated. Your agent will guide you as to what looks best on film vis-à-vis your mode of dress, the actual pattern of your clothing, your color scheme, and the kind of clothes that your portrayed character is supposed to be wearing. Your makeup and hair will also have to be suited to the character role. Try to feel comfortable with your costume, so that you can concentrate on the critical part of the audition.

You will arrive at the audition site at the scheduled time, tell the receptionist that you are there, and then wait, nervously sizing up the competition. You will have brought your resume and your head shot, which you will leave for the casting director to review or merely to remind him or her who (of the thousands) you were.

After a while, you will be introduced to other models who may be sharing this commercial with you. You will also be given your script and told the general story line of what will be acted in your little scenario. You may or may not have a speaking part. If you do speak, you will have to memorize your lines as well as the cues and directions.

Suppose you are trying for a hair product commercial. Directors usually look for blonds, because highlights are more easily picked up when the hair is light, and because the United States is a blond-oriented society. Semilong hair has more movement to it and is considered to be more sensual. If you have both the right color and length, your chances are greatly improved. Your next problem is to move with ease and be completely relaxed with a television camera, crew, and a whole roomful of strangers with your miniskit jiggling around in your head.

Having gotten this far, you are ready to go in front of the cameras. Things seldom go as planned. You may find yourself doing not one but as many as a dozen or more takes. If there are more people involved in the commercial, it could take quite a while just to coordinate everyone. Trying to make each take seem fresh and natural is easier said than done. Take number one may be stiff, but by the time you get to take number fifteen, exhaustion will have overcome stiffness.

If you can develop the knack of doing television commercials, the thousands of dollars plus residuals paid for each one more than compensate for the boredom, anxiety, cattle-call degradation, and myriad takes.

After successfully getting through one of these little commercial vignettes, you may consider doing another one. Viewers automatically assume that if a person endorses a product (models with it or promotes it verbally), that person surely *uses* it as well. This is often just not the case, but the manufacturer of the product that you have promoted does have the right to prevent you from modeling for that company's direct competitors for a period of time (depending on the contract you signed). If you modeled for a certain company's new color-rinse shampoo and then were offered a commercial by another hair product company to model their antidandruff shampoo, the advertisers would see that as a definite conflict of interest. You will be financially compensated to turn down the second company's offer. You could, however, model any unrelated area of products from any nonshampoo-making company.

If you don't land that first commercial, try again. If you believe that your hair is your best asset, try out for all the endless hair accessories, hair dryers, shampoos, rinses, dyes, clippers, pins, gels, curling irons, hair pieces, treatments, medications, highlighters, curlers, home permanents, and even stylists' commercials. Hairdressers' competitions have helped some models later obtain a hair commercial. Several known models got started with just such a TV commercial.

Unions

Unions strictly protect people who perform in the commercials, monitoring pay scale, time allowed to work, and where and when work can be done. When you try for your first commercial, you will not need to worry about unions; you are permitted one "free" commercial before you are forced to join a union (or unions). The union sets a uniform pay scale that must be strictly adhered to regardless of the person's status as model, actor, or even person off the street. All ages of people are included in these codes. Your agent can advise you as to which unions to join and where and how to pay your annual dues.

There are two unions that you may need to join if you intend to do extensive work in television commercials. One covers live commercials and the other covers videotaped commercials:

AFTRA
  (American Federation of
    Television and Radio
    Artists)
  260 Madison Avenue
  New York, NY 10016

SAG (Screen Actors' Guild)
  1515 Broadway
  New York, NY 10036

There are rules as to which union coverage you will have to have. Lacking an agent, you must be responsible for your own protection. That means inquiring and applying for these union memberships as needed.

Membership in the American Federation of Television and Radio Artists (AFTRA) is currently $1,000 and annual dues are $42.50 semiannually. AFTRA is an open union.

Membership in the Screen Actors' Guild (SAG) is currently $1,160.50 and annual dues are $85, plus 1.5 percent over $5,000.

To apply for membership to the guild, you must have done anything under SAG's jurisdiction (such as a screen feature film or commercial) or have been a member of one of the following for at least a year:

AEA (Actors' Equity Association)
AFTRA (American Federation of Television and Radio Artists)
AGMA (American Guild of Musical Artists)
AGVA (American Guild of Variety Artists)
Hebrew Actors' Union
Italian Actors' Union

Resume

A resume is very important if you are planning to audition for television commercials. The resume should give all the critical statistics. A particular style or layout, clever arrangement of the critical information, or artistic touches may help you catch the employer's eye. The most important thing is to remember that your resume's function is to include all of the pertinent data and make a neat impression. Therefore, the first section must include your name, address, and phone number (or that of your answering service, manager, or agent).

The next section should include your social security number and your union associations and membership numbers.

The following section should include your physical data: height, weight, hair color, eye color, and your general look or type. Include the age range that you could honestly portray. Your clothing sizes should be listed—for a suit, shirt, shoe, hat, and gloves if you are a man; and for a hat, dress, shoe, glove, and undergarments and swimwear if you are a woman. Most women are more detailed in the department of measurements. You may want to be explicit as to bust, waist, and hip measurements.

As you will be promoting your vocal abilities if you intend to talk (and talking in any commercial doubles your pay scale) in your audition and subsequently in commercials, you will want to mention the level of your voice (tenor, for example) and the list of any movies or commercials you've done. Mention any live theater productions and the parts you acted. Give all the correct information about each theatrical production, including where and when it was performed.

If you were coached by someone of renown, list it clearly under *Professional* or *Special Training.* Also indicate any dance training, fencing, competitive sports, or any other type of movement instruction that could indicate agility or skilled grace. Mention any kind of unusual talent or skill—like sky-diving, scuba diving, windsurfing, sailing, skiing, diving, ice-skating, horseback riding, pizza tossing, whistling.

The ability to speak any foreign languages should be noted, and your own nationality and native tongue if it is not simply North American. Even variations in United States accents can make or break your chances at the job.

One last thing to include in your resume is the name of a reference or two if you are not being represented by an agent upon introduction.

Your resume is most often typed on a sheet of paper that fits against and is firmly attached to your glossy eight-by-ten photograph, back to back. Nothing says that you have to fill up your eight-by-ten resume, but do center the information. Neatness and professionalism count a great deal. If you value your crack at the commercial, make your photograph and your resume attractively displayed and appealing.

The photograph that is so important is supposed to be a lively image with projection. The old high school graduate shot is considered to be too stiff and certainly won't get you past the casting agent. There is such a prescribed definitive look that you have to spend a good bit of time on this project. More often than not, your idea of how you look best is *not* their idea of your best shot! They want to see how you will come across as a warm, believable, likable person. This is not an easy request of one sample photograph.

After much stewing and brewing in front of a photographer who specializes in head shots for television commercial hopefuls, you may come up with one or even two passable shots. Try to get another professional opinion about which shots are best for you. The expense of these head shots will be $500 to $1,000, depending on your choice of photographer and how many prints you decide to have made. This can be a rather large investment if you are doing many auditions and you leave the photograph with attached resume with the casting directors of each. But this photograph can be the reminder that could and often has secured a future or even a different job than the one you tried for.

CHAPTER 4

OPENING THE DOOR TO MODELING

CAN MODELING SCHOOL HELP YOU?

Modeling schools were first established in the thirties and forties when professional modeling began to rise with product-association sales. John Robert Powers saw the need to educate the totally naive girl on how to present herself to the client as a desirable image to be copied by women and as a status symbol to a man. Hundreds of modeling agencies have since jumped on the bandwagon. In the smaller cities, you can find many a school-agency that introduces the totally green model to the basics of the business as well as gives the first work as the agent.

Modeling schools do not offer the promise of any success. Their job is merely to show a little of the inner workings of the profession. As far as becoming a model with or without a future, it is merely a chance endeavor on your part. It would be unfair to assume that the modeling school can make you into a model any more than any school can produce a graduate with a guarantee of success. Carefully investigate the benefits of the modeling school before you enroll. It could be a complete waste of money and time if the agency of your choice wants to provide its own instruction, leads, and guidance.

Depending on your actual limitations as far as modeling jobs, you may find it very beneficial to take a modeling school course that is given in conjunction with local contacts and known work.

Familiarity with how you appear on film and video can give you insight into your potential future in the varied areas of modeling. Mock-ups of actual "shows" will prepare you for work with commentators, as timing is an essential in this work. Every modeling situation will be different, but the more aware you are of what may occur, the more confident you may feel.

There are modeling schools in every major city where you could inquire about the courses given, the time allotted, and the cost. Some of the schools are strictly charm instruction and will simply give the student a little polish. In really rural areas, exposure to self-improvement courses is valuable simply as an introduction to basic fashion.

In very small towns, modeling work is generally limited to department store shows and social events where models might provide the entertainment for a ladies group. The school may work as a small agency and may or may not collect a fee to arrange these modeling shows. But the model is usually compensated in some way and at the very least is gaining experience and exposure to the public.

The reason for attending any school is to learn to do something that you did not know how to do beforehand. There are many hundreds of people who have all the raw qualities mentioned in Chapter 2. For people who already have great self-assurance and all the needed physical attributes, attending modeling school would be superfluous.

A modeling agency that wants to put you under contract though you are completely inexperienced will undertake your training or see to any needed instruction. Many agencies see to your development in a European arena because those photographers are better known for taking the time to work with a very young and inexperienced model.

With European training, it is easier to land the higher paying jobs in the United States. Some models become enamored with not only the modeling work in Europe, but with the lifestyle there. For many, what started as an education in a new field turned into a career in itself. Modeling in France, Germany, and Italy has been the highlight for many young models whose careers started there. (See Chapter 5 under "Modeling in Other Countries.")

The modeling school is an avenue by which you can glean a little polish, savvy, and a rough idea of the many areas of the work itself. The schools will not let you observe a class in session (as a rule). Therefore you will have to weigh your own abilities and decide whether you think that you would benefit from this type of school. If you know of someone who has attended a particular school and that person is willing to tell you about it, that might be very helpful.

Fees are commensurate with the area where the school is located, the curriculum, the actual facilities of the school, and the length of the courses taught. There is no guarantee that you will emerge as a model or even that you will get a single job as one.

What might an established modeling school really do for you, and what does it cost?

A school in a rural area gives modeling instruction, charm classes, pageant preparatory courses, and general self-improvement instruction.

The modeling course should include:

- posture, carriage, and walk
- diet, exercise, and figure control
- nail care
- skin care
- hair care and styling
- wardrobe coordination and fashion
- etiquette and social graces

Classes should familiarize the young person with all the terminology and some of the equipment needed for the modeling trade.

In the New York City area, the tuition for between forty-five and sixty hours of instruction would be about $1,200 to $1,600. Techniques for the various areas of work are stressed. In a very rural area, it is often through this one channel that the completely naive youngster gets started. One of the biggest models today was introduced to her profession through a modeling/charm school in the rural North-east. She was spotted by a teacher there who recognized her potential. She went through their program, armed with a small amount of self-assurance, and was then on to the big city. She was a supermodel in about a year's time.

So even if the outlay of the tuition is a bit of a gamble as far as your guaranteed return (no one can assure you of even one modeling job from your schooling), it can also be the leg up that will get you into the real arena. If you are totally unprepared for the eventuality of the work even in front of the camera, you just may miss out completely. There are no hard and fast rules on how to come from the rural or smaller areas and make a smooth transition into a trade that so obviously demands a real sense of sophistication and flair. Most natural beauties who are country lasses have a freshness that is very highly sought by the modeling agencies in all sectors of the modeling world, and they are usually happy to put the polish on the naive young lady themselves.

The experience for a prospective model is extremely limited in such areas, but original exposure for most models did not originate in New York City or Los Angeles. It is not too difficult to contact neighboring areas and send a letter requesting an interview at one or two of their agencies. Modeling usually pays a high enough wage to make it worth your while to travel a bit for that necessary exposure. You have to be seen to be in demand, and in modeling you have to make every effort to be noticed in the best way possible.

In larger cities, like Atlanta, Cleveland, San Francisco, and Boston, modeling schools are more visible. Some of these schools have associated agencies that help students find work.

If there are more modeling jobs available through these particular school-associated agencies, you may seriously want to look into the school itself, even though you may not think that you really need the courses. In many middle-sized cities, modeling school classes are more comprehensive, simply due to the demand for more sophisticated modeling work. Thus the tuition is higher. Though it would be impossible to give an exact dollar value from city to city, the average seems to be around $1,200 for the basics.

A modeling school in New York City should be looked into as carefully as any other institution of learning. Merely the fact that it bears a New York City address does not guarantee that it is good. The sessions offered in most New York modeling schools cost between $1,300 and about $1,500 for the shortest curriculum in all-round modeling. The classes may be spread over as many as nine months or be as concentrated as one month. They are for both men and women and should include the basic knowledge needed to start with any agency. Help is given on how to handle your interviews at agencies, what pictures might be needed, and how to compile a resume.

If you are planning to go to New York City or Los Angeles, remember that your board and room can be astronomically expensive. You should make concrete inquiries and confirm reservations before your arrival.

If you are at all fearful of the legitimacy of a school or agency, inquire about it at the Better Business Bureau, an organization that can provide information on the business history and reputation of the school or agency in question.

PHOTOGRAPHS

Only a handful of people can simply step in front of a camera, not feel dreadfully inhibited, and get on with it. Just look through your family album to see those fishy stares while facing that terror—a camera.

An agent once said that after several months, models start to relax enough to be able to present themselves. There is something just dreadfully inhibiting about finding yourself a few feet away from that critical little eye of the camera's lens.

Most photographers try to elicit the right reactions from you with music, subtleties in voice, directions, and atmosphere. Some of the most interesting shoots are taken "on location"—where the product or the fashions would most likely be used. Usually, you get to film outside. It's not everybody's idea of fun—the wind, rain, heat, or freezing cold can put a damper on things.

The idea of feeling inhibited must be overcome before you will be able to do your best work in front of the camera. Many agencies in New York City that hire you will see to your development. That often means an internship in

Europe with many photographers. These photographers will teach you how to move, how to "freeze," and how to develop your own special attitude and "look" for the camera. They are known for being very patient and will work with you until they can get the correct look on film. The pictures are often quite beautiful and become part of the models' portfolios when they return here to continue their careers.

Another way to acquire photographs is to ask other models who did theirs. You can then call the photographer and ask if he or she is testing. If tests are arranged, the model takes the film and pays for processing. The photographer gets to pick from the slides. Both are responsible for their own printing. This benefits both parties, as both need shots for their portfolios. It is a very good way to make contact with as many good photographers as possible. The photographer is often the one who makes recommendations to the client, and that's a plus for you. If you are a good model for the photographer's work, he or she will be able to promote you.

Portfolio

The portfolio is the most important representation of a model and her or his work. Every time you have an appointment for a potential job, you must drop off your portfolio. The client then studies all of the types of photographs that you have displayed and decides whether you would be the perfect model for the work that will be photographed.

Portfolio photographs currently cost between $1,000 and $2,500 in New York City. Check with the agencies of your choice if you are planning on taking professional shots to interviews. Printing is costly and you should think ahead, or you may find yourself spending more money than you thought possible.

Most photographs using models are accompanied by the photographer's name, so if you find photographs in a style to your liking, you may want to contact that photographic studio. For television modeling, you have to have photographs going in. The head shots for this specialized type of modeling should depict you at your warmest and friendliest; your fashion photographs would be unsuitable.

Expect to pay $500 or more for a head shot for television commercials. This would be an 8 × 10 in black and white that you would have printed and leave at all the "possible jobs," accompanied by your resume.

Many times when the selection is to be made, it is only your photograph in a two-foot deep heap of them that reminds the director who was even there. You can see how critical good photographs are to your potential work. There are also times when you may not be selected for the original job that you were seeking, but that photograph left on file has been pulled and gotten you another, totally unrelated job. One male model was very unhappy about missing out on a particular job, only to have been remembered by the director for his dramatic Japanese good looks. When his photograph was pulled several months later, he was handed not one, but three really fantastic accounts. His head shot had portrayed him in native Japanese costume while he, of course, appeared in impeccable western attire for his interview and screen test. The director could see how striking and versatile the model could be. He was just what they were looking for at that future time, and this model had surmounted the greatest hurdle for anyone going on a television audition. Get noticed, and then be the one and only one who's remembered. These casting directors see thousands of hopefuls every day, and there are many who are pretty much the same or could feasibly do the same commercial, so they are impressed with the uniqueness that you can project in the two minutes flat that you'll be viewed initially.

BEGINNING EXPENSES

If you are planning to move to New York City or Los Angeles, you will have to have a large nest egg to tide you over, unless you are planning on working at some other job while you try to break into modeling. The rent alone will probably be $1,000 per month, and that would be sharing a one-bedroom apartment with someone. Many models share their apartments with one or more models. The costs are so high that even studio apartments run $1,500 per month.

Food will be the next most expensive item in your budget. Food costs in New York City have doubled in the past few years. It used to be possible to save money by cooking at home; now food is so expensive that it is often just as reasonable to go to a neighborhood restaurant. At any rate, your food bill won't be less than $200 per week.

Transportation costs are rising steadily, too. New York City buses and subways are now $1.50 per ride, and taxis are about $4 a mile in the city, considering the heavy traffic.

Medical and dental expenses should be anticipated. You won't be able to fly back to Kansas when your filling comes out in an untimely crunch. A filling could cost about $300. New York City is really not a place to be caught without medical insurance coverage.

Add all of the above figures together, plus an allotment for personal items, entertainment, household items, telephone ($150 deposit), and gas and electricity, and you will have an idea of what it could cost you to live.

Add the cost of the photographs that you may initially need, the cost of your portfolio case itself ($100), your makeup (which will be extensive if you are a woman), clothing, and any sports gear that you might require. Nobody ever said that New York City was an inexpensive city to live in or that modeling was an inexpensive profession to get into. It is a game to juggle all of the figures; eventually you'll come up with your own solutions on how and where to save pennies.

A FEW HELPFUL HINTS

Due to the tremendous competition in the field of modeling, you will want to be as well prepared prior to your attempted launch into the modeling world as is physically possible. You cannot know exactly what may be the current trend, but you can get yourself in top condition.

Movement

Many agents complain that models who are very good in other areas do not move well enough. There is not only a knack to moving well, but the more trained you are at an early age, the more defined are the long slender muscles that are the trademark of the best-looking people. You must choose carefully what kind of exercise will give those extended lines. Ballet, gymnastics, swimming, and tennis are all very good forms of strenuous exercise that give the body a definitive shape. All of the foregoing are suggested in moderation; three to four hours a week would be ample. You do not want to develop an overabundance of muscle.

Wherever your natural forte lies is the best place to put your greatest effort. Many well-known fashion models are simply not graceful to the professional eye, yet they have enough going for them that they are top models. If you watch videos or actual fashion shows, you will see amazing variations in natural grace. Some people move with incredible ease, while others remain visibly uncoordinated throughout their lives.

You can make the best of either possible case by starting early to take some kind of regulated exercise and sticking with it. A child who starts to take dance lessons before he or she becomes inhibited about moving in front of peers will have a much better chance of overcoming awkwardness. If a child reaches the age of about seven and has never been encouraged to develop any natural abilities like swimming or playing ball, that child may well remain ill-at-ease with any request to move when a possible audience might see her or him.

Teeth

Take excellent care of your teeth! Your smile is a paramount introduction to you—not only for cosmetic reasons, but because bad teeth tell the world that you don't think enough of yourself to take care of them. The male model is primarily noted for his teeth (and his eyes). Men have to have a great smile to sell the product. Women models have to have pretty teeth as part of the whole picture.

Teeth can make or break your career as a model. Many real beauties do not have those perfect teeth and as a result photograph badly. Your teeth could be too far apart, too long, or too irregular. There are many ways to make the needed corrections, and not all of them are even permanent. One famous model uses a spacer between her two front teeth only when certain shots require that look. She often models au naturel, with her space between her front teeth as her very own trademark!

Makeup

Makeup is a critical factor for all women models. Applying makeup is an art. When you do a fashion shot, a makeup artist or stylist does your face. This can be as time-consuming as two hours or more. If you are doing catalog and other similar types of work, you will have to do your own makeup and do it well.

There are many tricks of the trade. Some of these can be picked up at places where makeup artists work on you, advise you as they go along, and show you how to bring out your best features. You are expected to buy makeup, but you also will pay for the makeup artists' work. Shading and highlighting are two of the most important things that you have to learn.

To do your makeup really well, you must understand what the camera sees and try to correct any flaws that nature has given you. If you have circles under the eyes, for example, you will want to use a small amount of moisturizer and cover those areas lightly with powder. This is a hard area to disguise and the less done the better. As you get older, less and less makeup is used. Heavy makeup only attracts the eye to the deepened facial lines, and the camera is very quick to pick up on all the imperfections accented by bad makeup.

In using makeup, you will discover the difference between what is worn in front of the camera versus what is worn in natural light. There are many tricks that involve shading. Dark colors make the object recede or seem less prominent, while light colors bring the object forward.

Lips, cheeks, and noses are all treated in special ways to make the best possible presentation. It will take you a while to gain the knack of how to handle all those makeup brushes, bottles, blends, cakes, pastes, and wands, but time will make you adept. Eventually you will be confident with your own ability to make your face look its best.

Fingernails

Your fingernails don't always need to be painted, but they have to be perfectly manicured. That means they should be really scrubbed, with no visible cuticle, and either coated with clear polish or buffed to a soft shine. Your nails are right out there, and there is no way to hide a lack of care on your part. Become adept with the emery board, and be able to keep both hands looking neat. Once you've started to make an income as a model, you'll want to head straight to the manicurist and the pedicurist once a week. The pedicurist will do to your feet what the manicurist does to your hands. These services together cost about $40 plus tip.

Legs

Leg waxing is critical for a model and is done on an as-you-need-it basis. Most women go to the salon at least once every six weeks, but if you are averse to all this time-consumption you may desire removal of hair from bikini line, legs, mustache, underarms, and eyebrows by electrolysis. In the long run it could save you money and time.

Fashion Sense

Try to develop your fashion sense as soon as possible. Exposure to art classes, sewing courses, and familiarization with costumes in museums and libraries are all helpful. You are not normally expected to create any of your ensembles for actual modeling work, but your own fashion sense will be valuable in your presentation of the clothing in front of the camera and in your presentation of yourself.

If you are paid to be a model, you are expected to look like one. That doesn't mean loads of makeup and thousand-dollar ensembles, but it does mean being clean and neat and giving a certain amount of care to your appearance. You never know whom you may meet, and a model has to be an opportunist. Often a job is offered when you least expect it. Not all jobs are found through go-sees. You are your own best advertisement, and the sooner you prepare yourself for self-sell, the better. So much of modeling is based on merely your looks that the best presentation possible can only help you.

Performance

Acting lessons, speech lessons, and voice instruction may be very helpful if you are aiming toward television work as part of your modeling profession. Any plays having a possible part for you should be given serious preparation and an audition.

Every experience that you could possibly have before an audience—choral singing, plays, variety shows, beauty pageants, and even attending social functions—can be helpful in giving you that critical self-confidence. Poise is gained by experience. Though modeling can only be done well by the truly experienced model, your efforts to meet the public and feel at ease in front of lots of people can aid you tremendously when you are asked to "perform" before the cameras.

If you wait until you are actually offered an audition for a television part to start to learn to speak well and dramatize a little, you probably will freeze and lose the part.

Many soap opera stars started as models and now enjoy much more financial security because they added the important talent of speech to their repertory of mime while they were still photographic models. Being prepared and being lucky enough to be there at the right time make the magical combination.

CHAPTER 5

MODELS' SALARIES

There are only two reasons to become a model: to be rich or famous, or both. Celebrity models have whizzed past the supermodel status. It is no longer enough to make those million-dollar salaries for those at the top of this field. Recognition and idol-worship have become the great salary boosters. It now costs a client stupendous amounts if the product is to be represented by a recognizably famous model. The cosmetic companies with their immense profitability are the big contracts to the models. Celebrity models are more often associated with makeup and fragrances than with any other products. Models who represent or are exclusive to one makeup or fragrance company may not represent another. However, they can accept other types of modeling jobs and are not restricted solely to that one company.

The average model can expect to earn commensurately with his or her locale and the advancement of client requests. Small-town models are often paid per job or a bit above minimum wage, while the more opportunity-filled big city can land you a salary of as much as $300,000 if you are working to capacity. The paycheck will reflect your rate of demand from a modest $15,000 to a pretty stunning bankroll of over a quarter of a million dollars, and these females are often only thirteen years old!

Runway work is usually paid at $150 per hour and could run a bit more or less depending on the time of year, the actual promoters, the number of models needed, and the size of the return expected from that showing. If the show is a very lavish one and continues for an extended length of time, that will be taken into consideration and the pay could run as high as about $250 per hour. Runway and fashion shows do not always have cash remuneration in the smaller cities, however, and pay may be made in clothing or even in makeup.

There are also photographic jobs available in moderation, depending on the size of the city and its prominence in the local fashion world. For the department store's advertising in the local newspapers and brochures, you could expect to be paid about $75 per hour.

Agencies in rural areas have a set rate for which the model may be hired. That rate would apply to whatever job the model might be requested to do, from live promotional work (where he or she might otherwise only make the doubled minimum wage) to photographic work. The agency might ask 20 percent, for example. This seems quite fair in that the agency then looks for better-paying jobs and you have a chance at developing a reasonable income. The idea here is that you would like to be a model *only* and not have to subsidize your income forever with other work.

Local manufacturers sometimes hire models for their showrooms. Such work, though seasonal, pays about $35 to $50 per hour. The work is only available a few weeks during the year, so you could not consider making a living from it.

In a middle-sized city where a model works at all of the aforementioned, there is simply not enough income available from modeling for you to have a real career of it. Ultimately, to make a career in modeling, you have to move to Chicago, Dallas, New York City, or Los Angeles. The experience gleaned in a smaller town will have given you a bit of self-confidence and will hold you in good stead. You will learn that having done your homework in any size city is what forms the basis of professionalism.

The high fashion industry is the only place where you can make a really full-time career as a model and be financially independent. This is true for both men and women. Though the male model could never hope to compete with a high fashion female model in salary or career, he could certainly make a sizable income in the fashion capitals.

Not long ago the top salaries for the fashion models in the middle-sized cities ranged from $8,000 to $12,000 a year. These were the best and the busiest models, and yet that was all the work that was available to them. Women in New York City who are just starting out with an agency are paid between $125 and $300 per hour depending on the kind of modeling. Male models in New York City have a starting pay of between $100 and $200 per hour depending on the agency. Some will and do pay up to $300 per hour.

The way to build up your hourly wage is by building up your popularity. The agency pushes their top models; if you work your way up to that category, you could be making the over-$300,000 salary. A particular look comes in, and if you are that look, your agency will capitalize upon it quickly. Fashion can be quite fickle. While you are the in look, you will have to move fast.

CATALOG WORK

There are many areas in which you could start reaping these salaries. The first area is known for its bread-and-butter support of models—catalog work. You've seen hundreds of catalogs stuffing your mailbox, especially around Christmas-time. The catalogs are distributed from department stores, mail order houses, food importers, sporting goods merchandisers, toy manufacturers, travel packagers, and many more. The companies hire models to demonstrate their wares or beam unself-consciously in everything from silk underwear to million-dollar furs and diamond necklaces. The more prestigious items will be modeled by the highest paid models. Though the salary may start at $187.50 to $250.00 per hour in the bigger agencies, your potential is really unlimited, and there are catalog jobs that are extremely well paid. If a model's fee is $500.00 per hour, and a client has that look in mind as the marketable face, that client knows what prestige a known model's face can bring to the product and its sales. It is becoming very popular to have a known rather than unknown face and figure—thus the constant search for new models who could become the coveted look of tomorrow. There is a similarity in the look of many of the known models, and though there is a professed trend to deviate from the tall-blond-and-leggy look, the demand from the clients still keeps them the highest on the want list.

The *editorial rate* for the high fashion models is generally pretty low. The current rate is around $150 per day starting pay. Editorial is the work that is print but not commercial like the actual promotion of a product such as soap or toothpaste. A model must do this kind of work in combination with commercial catalog work to survive. Generally speaking, any woman in high fashion could do catalog work, but many of the models that you see doing work in catalogs are not high fashion models. For catalog work, you generally do your own makeup; for fashion work, it is usually done for you.

You can tell by looking at the models if they are high fashion or not, and looking should be part of your preparation for a modeling career. Scan the material that comes your way for the qualities of the fashion model. Your eye will become accustomed to a certain polished look and demeanor. You won't be able to distinguish this by what they are promoting or what they are wearing, but by the stance, projection of attitude, and "feel" of the model.

The more projection the model has, the better the look of that person will be remembered, and that's what will make the hourly rate skyrocket.

You will want to do a mixture of both catalog work and fashion work. Catalog is the bread and butter of modeling work, as the pay scale is good ($187 to $250) per hour; but without fashion work, you won't hold your own in the industry. So you must have a good balance of these two types of work to remain a photographic model represented by an agency.

You are of course paid for your time while you are being made up, having your hair styled, and having the clothing fitted before a photographic session.

RUNWAY WORK AND FASHION SHOWS

There are some high-paying and some rather moderate rates for the same type of work. Runway work that is done in various hotels for business groups and some social functions is occasionally done by models just starting in the field, some fresh out of a modeling school. The models are offered this experience in exchange for photographs and are not remunerated in cash. The photographs and the experience itself are both very valuable to the inexperienced model.

Informal modeling in department stores in New York City is on a pay scale of about $100 per hour. These are the models who do the fashion work in everything from expensive gowns to bathing suits in the largest stores. They are always exceedingly thin but not necessarily photogenic.

Big fashion shows could pay as little as $250 to $500 per hour. The model is compensated at half that pay while being fitted. The fees can go much higher than the aforementioned rates. One Seventh Avenue showroom pays $300 per hour for runway work. Depending on where it is in the world and where the show lies in the fashion season, more or less will be paid.

If you choose to work for a showroom on Seventh Avenue as a model, you will gain experience but not get paid a great deal. This is a weekly job with a weekly salary. Some models like the security of the nine-to-five job, but the difference in your potential salary is significant. The weekly salary would vary according to your experience and the type of garments that you are required to wear.

Much of Seventh Avenue does not require a high fashion model, and there is work to be found there even if you are as short as five feet, six inches. You need only be moderately attractive and pleasant in personality, as you deal directly with customers. You could be modeling any garment from junior sportswear to bathing suits. Current weekly salaries for the huge variety of Seventh Avenue models can be found in the want ads in the local papers. Pay in the smaller department stores is currently about $60 per hour.

Go to several interviews if you plan to work on Seventh Avenue or in the department stores. It will give you an idea where you will fit in best. Both are live modeling jobs, and both could potentially lead to other things. The main difference is the figure type required. The Seventh Avenue model *could* be the shorter, bustier woman. The department store model who shows women's clothing will have to be at least five feet, eight inches or taller and weigh less than 120 pounds. Some Seventh Avenue models will have the high fashion prerequisites also. If this seems a bit confusing, it is because the garment district has very different needs in its models than high fashion alone.

All you would have to do to get a clearer idea of who might be modeling on Seventh Avenue is to wander through the endless sections of junior to large-size clothing in the stores. If a garment is sold, it was probably modeled for a buyer at some point. The way to narrow the field is to read the specifications in the daily want ads that are calling for models for the garment section.

A whole group of models—women over five feet eight inches tall and weighing 150 to 200 pounds—has come into demand. Such women are needed by the market to model the clothing that a vast number of women now need. Not only are more women taller than they ever were, but they are proportionately filled out. These models can find work not only on Seventh Avenue, but also in photographic work to sell the large-size clothing. The salary level here could be more than $200,000, potentially, per year. Everything from large-sized swimming suits to evening gowns needs to be modeled, so there are plenty of jobs available in this area. Not all agencies handle the large-size model, but you would definitely want to be handled by an agency to guarantee the highest income, unless you wanted to start in the garment district where you would be a weekly salaried employee.

A good model who has just started out should not expect to make anything for the first three months. After that, the jobs should start coming in and the model should reasonably expect to have at least three jobs a week. By the beginning of the second year, you should be making at least $50,000, and from then on the sky is the limit. You will bring in just as much as you yourself are willing to work for. There are always appointments to go to. If you are enthusiastic and have the needed look, you'll be out there perhaps six or seven times every day on "go-sees." No one who has worked as a model could ever call it anything but very hard work!

The model who pushes constantly could certainly see a salary above $250,000.

You will want to do jobs with as much variety as possible to take advantage of your youth. Remember that this career cannot last past the age of twenty-three, unless you are extremely lucky and your face shows no lines. So you have to work extra hard every day, make absolutely certain that you really want this so badly that you're willing to give your all, and you're sure to make it!

With a good agency behind you, and the two of you cooperating on your career, you might just become one of the million dollar models! You'll never know unless you get out there and explore the field. You have to start early. Right now is not too soon!

MODELING IN OTHER COUNTRIES

Modeling in Europe as a way of entering the field is becoming more and more popular. When you are signed by an agency, an apprenticeship (period of learning) in Europe to work with fashion, makeup, photographers, and methods of handling yourself and paraphernalia usually lasts about six months. At that time, most fashion models return to their agencies in the United States. If you should be lucky enough to land some paying work in Europe, you could find yourself working in England, Sweden, Denmark, Belgium, France, Holland, Germany, or Italy. If you decide to return to any of these countries at a later time, you will probably find enough modeling work to keep you happy while you enjoy Europe as well.

There are of course many "on location" jobs where an American model or several models are sent to work. These stays are not lengthy, and many models complain that they have been places but had so little time to sightsee that they don't know anything about where they were. At some point in your career, you may want to relocate. The money to be made in modeling is excellent worldwide.

The Japanese market is opening ever wider to Western models. Many young models have been there to do commercial and editorial work. Many catalogs and brochures have featured American models in exotic lands and countries. Many American models who have relocated for any length of time live in Europe.

EXCLUSIVE CONTRACTS

Most models hope for an exclusive contract with a company whose product they are hired to represent in every type of media possible. The people who first come to mind are those women whose faces have been the sole (or almost sole) model for the huge cosmetic companies. Exclusivity means that the model will only be photographed in that company's cosmetics. This prohibiting act (on the part of the company) is very expensive for the client. By cutting off the model's other possible sources, the hiring company contracts her at a fee that must satisfy her and compensate for all the other potential work that she might have been able to do. Exclusivity is so highly paid that most models are very desirous of such an arrangement. The best part of this type of contract is of course the security and the fame that come with being associated with some of the most prestigious products. Exclusive contracts have been known to go to $1,000,000 per year, and every year these star jobs get even higher dollar fees.

INEXPERIENCED VERSUS
EXPERIENCED MODELS' FEES

The fees indicated in this chapter for the various types of modeling are all the bottom rates. As a model becomes more well known and is more in demand, the agency will raise her or his fee. It works somewhat like the supply and demand in any business. The model's fees keep increasing and level off when the demand does. The demand could just stop altogether, too, so one has to be prepared for many eventualities.

Always be prepared for the best *and* the worst. No one can predict the future. Some of the women and men who looked like they were going to set the world on fire, within a month, fizzled almost instantaneously.

Experienced models' fees, if all goes well, are often more than $300,000 per year.

The lucky and very rare model whose career takes flight instantaneously could make that half million dollar salary or more! Only one lucky model in ten thousand will make it at all, and the ratio is even greater—much greater—for supermodels.

The models who are making such high yearly salaries are combining many forms of modeling—high fashion, runway, television, catalog, editorial work, videos, and even posters. The money to be made from all of these sources collectively is stupefying!

While the model has a look that is salable, the money must be made and quickly. Youth does not wait, and popularity can and does wane, so the clever model makes all the money possible during her halcyon days.

CHAPTER 6

AGENTS, AGENCIES, AND MANAGERS

With the tremendous frenzy of model wanna-bes, the whole thrust of modeling agencies has shifted. It is almost as if the agencies are smothered with resumes, appointments, and bodies at open calls. Agencies have always needed to have rosters of varied models for the prospective clients to select from, but with the tremendous influx of desirous models, they are in the catbird seat. It used to be most advantageous for models to look around at what each and every different agency could possibly offer them. Now it is all you can hope for if at least one agency takes a serious interest in you.

At one time it was possible to freelance by using small agencies, contacts, and referrals. Today, if you don't have an agency behind you, you're sure to get lost in the hordes.

The ideal would be to have an agency represent you that would take you on and send you to at least several go-sees per day. With the current status, there are many models who could be the perfect one for the client, so it is just that much more difficult to become established.

Small agencies are able to push you a bit more but may not have the bigger clients, while the large and more established agencies have many more models to choose from who may take some of the potential work from you. Also there are certain styles and characteristics of all the better-known agents. Often the youngsters sink or swim due to the mentoring relationship of their agents. They have a vested interest in you as you will be the one making the fees that keep the agency afloat. You pay them the normal 20 percent and the client pays them as well. So there are many reasons to have as good representation as is possible.

You may be thrilled that an agency has agreed to take you, but if you feel that you are not being handled to your best advantage, you can always consult those who have been there and then go on. In the past, some of the bigger models in particular have sought their own personal managers to guide their tremendous financial contracts. Agents, like all others, can be wonderful, or not so wonderful. Personal agents are only as good as the return they can get for the both of you.

SELECTING THE RIGHT AGENCY FOR YOU

It is up to you to choose the agency that you think could use your particular look to the optimum. Every agency specializes in a certain style. Familiarize yourself with the various models that each agency represents. You will see the similarities in their overall look, and you must then judge where you think you fit in best.

Weigh the advantages and the disadvantages of the smaller versus the larger agency prior to calling for an appointment. A smaller agency would more than likely be able to get you more work, but its pay scale could be as low as half of what you could make at one of the bigger agencies! One tremendous advantage to working for a smaller agency is that if you are completely green, you will gain experience and become polished in the interim.

The bigger agency is in a better position to pay the larger fees to models. Your pay scale could be doubled with a large agency. However, though you may be sent on nearly twice the number of go-sees as the smaller agency could send you on, the larger agency has more models for that same client to interview for the same job.

After you have made an appointment for an interview at the agency of your choosing, you will start the process of making what you hope will be the perfect match.

At that all-important interview, let the interviewer do the talking. Listen carefully and answer all of the questions as concisely as you can. Most of the questions will be to establish your height and measurements and to get a reasonable understanding of what you expect from the modeling world and how you think that the agency will fit into the scheme of things.

Questions like "Why do you want to model?" and "Why do you think that you would be good at it?" are just two of the things they'll be likely to ask. Remember that they can be very personal, and you should be prepared to take personal questions in stride.

At your interview do not be modest, but do not brag either. Any extra talent that the agency may be able to promote for you is money in both your pockets. If you are a good athlete, dancer, skin diver, or even were in many serious dramatic productions, be sure to mention it at your interview. There are many occasions where a model is required to show off ski gear, and it may not be from a chairlift alone! Don't exaggerate when it comes to your actual ability. You may get caught in your own little deception and find yourself at the top of the hill with all the cameras on you *waiting* for you to actually ski down!

No one can tell you beforehand if you will be hired by any agency; on the other hand you may be offered a contract within minutes of your interview. Be prepared for both possibilities. You cannot take the lack of an offer as a personal rejection, as the interviewer may honestly believe that you might fit in better somewhere else, in which case to hire you would be a disservice to both of you. If an interviewer sees no future in creating a business relationship, you must take it as a positive statement and simply look into another agency. It is less likely that you will have to go to more than one interview if you genuinely try to understand *who* are the types of models that each agency represents. One very pretty young woman worked in an agency for a few months; having been employed in their office, she then set out to try the modeling end of things. She got up her courage, sized up all of the agencies, selected the one she thought best for her, and she was hired on the spot. Working on the inside for a summer gave her the discerning judgment to know which agency she fit into.

Having been just hired by an agency, you cannot even imagine how much it can guide your destiny. It is up to the agency to send you where you can potentially perform at your very best for both of you. You are in business together, and though it may be able to open some doors, your own caliber of work and self-sell will have to keep those doors open.

An agency will sign you only if it believes that the contract will be mutually beneficial. This means that the agency will do everything in its power to promote you, to get auditions and interviews lined up for you, and to make you into a more salable look. Therefore, it is of paramount importance that you and your agency be not only compatible but really honest and straightforward with one another.

Fees

The agency must set your fees wisely for the various types of work that you will be doing. The agency will set up your go-sees, and it is up to you to give it all you've got—to get to the appointment on time looking great, make the right impression, and present your book and yourself as professionally as possible.

The agency is there to protect you. Once it has set your fees and you have done a job, the agency will bill the client and collect your fee. You are responsible to your agency for a percentage of your fee for services rendered. There are no set percentages, but you can expect to have your agent charge 20 percent. That seems to be the usual rate, but some agents charge per big contract. Be certain that these things are spelled out clearly in your contract.

THE AGENT'S JOB

The agency is your answering service, business manager, bookkeeper, secretary, advisor, tutor, and even your guide as to weight reduction, hairstyle, makeup, and diet.

The agency protects you from unscrupulous clients and unprofessional people with whom you may come in contact. A model does not have to accept a particular job if he or she does not wish to. The power of the agency can make it more difficult for less than legitimate contacts.

The agent sees to the right model selection for go-sees. It is his or her business to comprehend what the client wants, and that model will be dispatched. It behooves the agency to have very clever people in its employ for discretionary selection. If agents judge incorrectly, a model from another agency gets the job.

When the agency sets up the go-see, the model is always advised about what to take to the particular appointment.

Frequently the garment to be worn is see-through or nearly so, and one wise model says that she never goes anywhere without bringing a bra, as she's found them required many times when the agency would never have thought of it.

Once under contract, you have to be sent on many go-sees to get started. If you are working in a small, slower agency, you could see three to four clients a day. A larger agency might send you on as many as seven or eight go-sees a day.

You will have only a few months; then if you do not start to "move," the agency may lose interest in you. Those first weeks are the make or break probationary time, so you have to convey your uniqueness, charm, and effervescence in a hurry.

If you are planning to move to a large city to work for an agency, it will often help you find housing. Ask your agent about this possibility if you are going to have to relocate to work.

Agencies are divided into different divisions if they handle large numbers of men, women, children, and a variety of television, runway work, and shows. There is so much complex work involved that it would be next to impossible to cope with the needs intelligently without having the various sections. Most models take advantage of as many kinds of work as their agency can offer them.

Many models feel that you are not taken as seriously if you try to freelance (work without being represented by any agent). A city like New York is so big that unless you have many personal contacts and know all the ropes, you are likely to find it nearly impossible to operate as a freelance model. The major benefit to being a freelance model is that you would not have any agency fees to consider in your budget. But if you cannot *get* any modeling jobs without the aid of the agents, then, of course, you have saved half of nothing.

Zed Cards

Most big agencies help defray expenses for your composites by supplying Zed cards. These are rather small cards with several photographs of you arranged in some sort of fashionable array. The composite is made of several of your selected photographs and is left as your calling card at the clients' when you have completed a go-see. This little card often gets you work at some future date, as the client can then open a file; though you may not have been perfect for the original job, you may be for subsequent ones.

Portfolios

Portfolios can be dreadfully expensive, and the book itself could cost $800. One roll could easily run $45 to $85, and you'll need at least ten to twelve different prints. By the time that you will have completed a good portfolio, it will have cost about $2,000. However, a good agency will help you build up your portfolio by "testing" (they send you to the photographers, and in return you and the photographer will each have prints) and spare you the cost of paying for the best photographers.

Your portfolio is extremely important. It is your most necessary tool of the trade. The clients must see how you look in print. The photographs in your book should give the widest range possible of your "looks" and allow the clients to have some insight into *how* you potentially will look in their commercial or print ad.

The agency should also help you to select the photographs that are the best ones for your portfolio. Its keen eye for what is good is honed through many years in the business, and its experience is financially valuable to both of you.

Control

An agency has a great deal of control over whom you will or won't work with through its selection of the models sent on go-sees. A good agency behind you can literally make you, as opportunities are made available for you to work your way up the ladder. The agent sets up the critical connections, and you have to cement them. With a large amount of luck, pluck, and energy, you can make it in the modeling field. The hardest part is getting started. Now that you know that the agency has put its vote of confidence in you, the rest is up to you!

CHAPTER 7

UPSIDES AND DOWNSIDES
OF MODELING

The competition for the really high paying jobs in modeling has brought the profession to a new level, both for the astounding money to be earned and the ages of the models. You often find females as young as thirteen who are completely on their own in cities like New York, Paris, and Los Angeles. These models are often from tiny communities where trust and family values were honored. They now find themselves in the sink-or-swim world of professional modeling. Some of the more reputable agencies have addressed this issue by offering housing dormitory-style to some of their novice models. But too often a young girl on her own finds trouble in the form of unscrupulous agents, photographers, and others near the industry who see the weakness of the wanna-be model and will try to take advantage of the situation. Burned-out teenage girls are endless victims of the missed brass ring on the carousel of modeling. Some of the young male models are destroyed as well, but their numbers are many times fewer.

The successful females who have risen to the top are not without their own problems. Not unlike many professions, the big money is the opiate of the model; hooked and trying to find meaning in a totally illusionary world, she is addicted. If you can discipline yourself to use the earnings from modeling to further yourself in a more in-depth career, it is often more rewarding. If celebrity and big money are the ends in themselves, you may find that happiness is often elusive. With this in mind, and presuming that you are fairly realistic about modeling, the following are some of the day-to-day pros and cons of the trade.

No matter how glamourous the life of the professional model looks to the observer, it is still a very disciplined job. Modeling has been promoted as a luxurious style of stardom and has an aura of ease, fun, excitement, and instant prestige. It has truly been the path to super riches and status for a few super models annually. It is often that promise of success and popularity that entices the young to seek modeling careers. Hearing from the models themselves gives a bit of insight into the realities of the daily down-to-earth work.

THE ADVANTAGES

- "The money is terrific. Nobody would *think* of paying me the kind of money that I make as a model, so I plan to stick with it as long as I can."
- "The best part is getting to go 'on location' because it's usually somewhere pretty exotic, and it was out of the

question that I'd ever get to see any of these places before I got to be a model. I've been to Italy and Japan, and Greece is a possibility."

- "Just having been a model for as long as I have been was an experience that no one could take away from me. It was kind of an education in itself."
- "It does have a lot of prestige in certain circles, and the contacts are great."
- "Some people think that it's a pretty glamorous job, and I agree with them! My lifestyle is so different now."
- "I love wearing all the beautiful, and some pretty weird things, too. It's theater on its own level."
- "I just happened to be lucky. My girlfriend and I started out together, and even though she is really a beauty naturally, I'm the bigger success because I wanted it so much more."
- "You get a lot of self-confidence from working as a model. Between the rejection and the praise it can be a little much, but it keeps you going if your head is where it should be. I know that I'm a good model and that it's hard work. It gives me self-satisfaction."

THE DISADVANTAGES

- "You always have to promote yourself. Your agency sends you out on a go-see, and the rest is up to you."
- "You always have to be 'up,' and even after days of being told that you're not the person for that particular

job, you *can't* let yourself feel dejected. It's all part of the game."

- "You never know how long a client will want you to represent the product. It's a real day-to-day risk."
- "I never can eat whatever I'd like. I have to think of the deprivation tomorrow if I have pizza tonight."
- "The hardest thing is that I can't go out to parties. I really have to be in bed early, and it really shows up on the camera if you haven't had at least eight to nine hours of sleep."
- "I'm really torn between continuing my modeling and getting a degree that I know I'll need very soon. The money is great right now, but I'll have to be behind all my friends if I put off my college until later."
- "It's hard to be in a profession where you know that you'll be a has-been by the time you're twenty-two."
- "It really is extremely hard work, and everyone who's never modeled somehow thinks that the end result was gotten by my standing around looking pretty."
- "I think that I really miss my sense of privacy most. That is the price you pay for notoriety."
- "You just have to be there at the right time. It's been really frustrating!"
- "The stress is incredible! I feel guilty if I'm tired."
- "Go-sees are really nerve-racking. It would be great to get all of your work through recommendation."

- "New York is a hard market to crack. You have to be a strong person. It's a vicious business, and you have to sift through it. You have to see it for what it is."
- "You have to provide your clothing. They do not give you the clothes that you model. That's just not true."
- "The fact that you never know that you will definitely have work worries me. I want to know that I'll be able to meet my bills. So many of us are out there now."
- "It's the kind of work where you just don't meet anyone to date. My hours and the fact that I work with mostly women can make life a little lonely."
- "The worst part for me is seeing how great the more seasoned models' books are. It'll take me a long time to get my photographs up there."
- "The discipline is really rigid. I wish that I could take a break from my diet, exercise program, and daily schedule, but if I'm not visible, there are just so many other girls who are dying for the work that I can't relax!"
- "My boyfriend accuses me of being self-centered. I know that modeling is a twenty-four–hour job, and if I don't watch out for my future jobs, nobody else will. We fight a lot about how much time my work takes me away from our relationship, but I really want to model, and I hope that we can stay together, too."
- "Sometimes the jobs are really boring. I try to pretend that they aren't by thinking of other things, but you have to keep your mind on what's going on so that you're

responsive. It's only good when you're getting a variety of work, and that doesn't always happen."

- "I find that New York is so unhealthy compared to my native state, and I would give anything to be able to have my career in modeling back in the Midwest. I know that's just impossible, but I'll stick it out here for a while longer because the money is so unbelievable."

- "It's hard to put up with some of the temperaments of the designers, stylists, and even some of the other models, but personality conflicts can be a problem in any line of work."

CHAPTER 8

AFTER YOUR MODELING
CAREER IS OVER

Modeling as well as its bosom buddy—fashion—are notoriously fickle. You could be shelved after just one or two seasons of success in clinching that quarter of a million in modeling work. Stunned and ego-bruised, you're a has-been at seventeen! Having left school to pursue the gold at the end of the runway, you'll now scramble to reassess your career. It is shocking to discover that your rising star plummeted mid-arc! However, if you were levelheaded enough to know that your very overinflated income was never guaranteed, then you prepared for this day all along. Don't ever let your ego convince you that the volatility of your profession makes any exceptions. No model is unsinkable, not even the supermodels.

With this in mind, do consider your next career during your venture into the modeling world. It always is certain that you will need another form of livelihood during your lifetime; it's just a matter of when. Granted, it will be a difficult transition to any real job after the big bucks from modeling, but try to invest some of that money so that you can enjoy as good a financial level as possible for many years after the modeling career has dimmed.

RELATED WORK

The type of work most frequently sought by models when their modeling careers are waning is in the field of *acting.* This is a natural sort of extension, in that you are still working in front of cameras, still being the ham. The major difference is you have to have or develop acting ability. Many models have tried this route only to discover that they fizzled as actors and actresses. Others are still out there in the public eye doing everything from videos to full-fledged Hollywood movies. They were smart enough to use modeling as a stepping-stone and made the connections needed while they were models. Television commercials prepared many of them with the knowledge of how to handle auditions and with the self-confidence and experience needed to cross over into movies.

Movie starlets are rarely acting wizards. Most of them are extremely attractive, so with a little luck the acting ability can be perfected on the way up. It is paramount that you photograph well, and you have that under your belt from the modeling experience. If you were or are a successful model, your chances of getting a part in a film are reasonable.

You have to follow your own desires when you are seeking another job. Though movies, television- or Hollywood-style, are in the offing, don't just take them because some-one *else* thinks that they are a terrific career. There are many types of work that you could do happily and well, so look around.

PHOTOGRAPHY

If you really are enthralled with fashion, there are many possibilities in conjunction with this area. Some models have made excellent *photographers,* because they under-stand something of the work after years in front of the lens. The creativity in this field has been fascinating to some models. A wide field of work could come from your endeavors.

Photography is very competitive and pretty much a self-sell occupation, much like modeling. The income to be made from this profession would depend on your choice of location, but if you pick a fashion center like New York City or Los Angeles, you could expect to start at $35,000. Good fashion photographers make salaries many many times that amount on an annual basis.

You may want to apprentice yourself to a photographer for a while and learn all of the inside tricks of the trade. As an assistant you won't make much money, but it may be the best way to enter the field.

There are several other areas of work that are involved with the photographic world, from stylist to makeup artist.

The *stylist* is responsible for the "look" to be created on the model. The hair, clothing, makeup, mood, and composite of the entire picture falls to the stylist. A real fashion sense comes into play here. You would put all of your past experience to work and be creative as well.

FASHION WORK

Fashion coordinators do work for department stores, fashion shows, and the like. Their work entails putting together clothing ensembles from shoes upward. There are many ensembles put together by fashion coordinators that are eventually the way the outfits become worn on the street or as a special costume.

Fashion designers are another whole group of fashion-conscious men and women—the core of the business. The designers create the look, and the model and the press carry it to the outside world. Fashion design entails an awareness of art, pattern making, the ability to sew (enough to understand *how* the pattern is going to fit), color coordination, marketing, and promotion.

This is a pretty tough field to tackle, but you may really love the area. In that case you will need schooling at a fashion institute and a great deal of luck. This is a very competitive and overcrowded field. Many start in it, but many drop out due to the number of talented people already in it.

If you have any writing talent, you may want to go into the editorial end of fashion. *Beauty editors* are often women who were or could have been fashion models and who have that sixth sense of what makes fashion and how to describe it to the public. Many fashions are presented to the world on the written page. These are not only exciting but also key jobs in the fashion world.

Some Seventh Avenue fashion models go directly into the *retail business,* as the work that they are involved in often includes sales. There are commissions to be made in this area, and if you are adept at sales, you may want to consider retail. Sales is the area that is currently opening to women at the fastest pace. There are several ways that you could stay in the fashion world with retail work.

Promotion and sales of every possible product in the fashion world could be handled by women. They understand the product and are excellent at the sales end of it. One of the biggest markets outside of the clothing industry is the makeup industry. This is another huge area in which women excel. Many directors of beauty and fashion are women, and some are former fashion models. Who could be more qualified than a beautiful woman who understands what women aspire to be?

When a fashion model leaves her chosen field of modeling at an age somewhere in her early twenties, she is at the prime point in her life to take responsibility for a decision-making job. She certainly will have had much experience in discipline, self-sell, fashion awareness, and competition along with a healthy dose of maturity. All of these traits are tremendous assets for the beauty industry to utilize. The wisdom of what makes fashion and beauty is the ongoing interest of the field. The women and men who were involved in one area of the fashion job market have often circulated to other areas and enriched all the facets of fashion in so doing.

Fashion illustrators are another critical group in the fashion world. As a model you may have sat for these artists. Their contribution is one of the stylized trademarks of the printed fashion world. Their work can be viewed everywhere, from museums to the daily newspapers. This is a very competitive field, one that employs a fine art.

Art school and a good bit of natural talent are the criteria. Some models have made it in this field, as some of them started out as illustrators and switched to modeling while the chance was offered. The four-year fashion school is the usual channel for entering fashion illustration; that schooling could run concurrently with your modeling career.

As the third largest industry in the United States, the fashion business has myriad job possibilities, and you'll want to put this foremost in your mind during your modeling career. The contacts that you make while you are modeling could be extremely helpful in your pursuit of future areas of work. Keep the contacts in mind, and keep their business cards as references in case you are interested in that particular area of work.

CAREERS FOR MEN

For male models, the decision will not be so critical. Male models who are successful can continue to work long into their late-middle years if they so desire. There are male models who have never had to seek another type of work and have lived well on their modeling incomes their entire adult lives. The fact that many major modeling agencies have expanded to accommodate male model divisions testifies to the fact that the men have really made their own mark in a once totally female-dominated world.

Male models who want to leave the field of modeling for various reasons (not the least of which could be lack of work) could easily fit into the sales end of fashions. Their fashion awareness would hold them in good stead, and the money to be made is substantial. Many men go into design from modeling work, as they have learned *what* is needed and desirable to the market. Many innovative styles are initiated by models. Much of the fashion world overlaps, and it is not surprising to see the needs of one area fulfilled by the intuitiveness of another.

CHAPTER 9

STARTING YOUR OWN MODELING AGENCY OR SCHOOL

Entrepreneurial models have often been the trail blazers in forming a new school or agency. Their familiarity with the profession gave them the insight into its shortcomings and how to build a better mousetrap. The combination of a past great model and a business partner is often seen. Business acumen is critical to the success of any endeavor, and you need only to look at the tremendous turnover of modeling agencies in the Yellow Pages of many cities to see how iffy those agencies are.

Many years ago, an enterprising woman saw the need for organizing the many facets of promotional modeling done within the various department stores in New York City. No one had thought of using an agency, because promotional models could be supplied from the few who had experience in the field, and at that particular juncture, there were only a handful. Those models were to promote the product as well as model it. The market was expanding so rapidly that there simply weren't enough trained people to fill the need. The entrepreneur started to collect the names and telephone numbers of the women whom she knew had done a little modeling; she contacted some who she thought would suit the needs of the companies who would hire the models. Due to the demand being by the week or even by the day, her agency had a nice little business going in almost no time at all. The models merely registered and then were contacted when this sporadic work arose. There were dozens getting work through this agency daily, whereas everyone without an inside connection had to scramble around looking for work through the manufacturer's offices every Monday. It really was a great idea; it benefited models and the companies that needed these particular models on short notice. The fees were usually a small percent of the daily income, as almost all of this type of promotional live modeling was and is paid by the hour. This particular agency is the simplest and least complex of them. The agent was continuing her work as a promotional model and supervising the agency as well. Specializing in a certain field worked for her because she knew that field very well.

This pattern has occurred repeatedly in people's transitions from modeling into owning agencies or managing models. The model who believes that he or she has a knack for business (and that is strictly what agents are all about) could put to use all the experience from the modeling years.

CREATING AN AGENCY

You will probably start with renting or buying some business space. If you plan to have several divisions within the agency, you will need a reasonable amount of space. If you intend to specialize, you can get by with as little as one room with a receptionist, secretary, booker, and you! The bare necessities are the needed equipment. How you attract your clients and models will be your most challenging problem, due to the intense competition.

You have to make certain that your chosen location will have the aura of chic, as that is the product that you are selling. If your office is too far from a high-class neighborhood, neither clients nor models will take you as being adept in your field. Organization is very important, too; you want to keep close track of your models and your clients.

If an agent isn't extremely busy, he or she will be out of business. Working on a percentage can be a pittance unless you represent hundreds of models on that percentage, and then you can be assured of more than a lovely income.

As a model who plans to enter the business world, you have to arm yourself with a completely different way of thinking. You will do well to take a few business courses and scan the general information in the course offerings from business schools. There are also advisory boards whose members are retired business executives. Their wisdom could guide you onto the right path without endless trial-and-error.

Financially, you will have to consider the rent, telephone, receptionist, bookkeeper, secretary or two, advertising, cost of furnishings, salaries of employees, taxes, many booking and telephone operators for your models and clients, and general office and business machines. You should visit an agency or two comparable to the type and size of the agency that you are planning. As a current (or past) model, you have a good idea of the inner workings of an agency, but if you've been working as much as most models, there are a lot of details that would have slipped by you. That was what *you* were paying your agent to do, to see to the smooth running of the agency so that you were free to do your end of the work.

Many modeling agencies in the large cities are located near one another. The most chic area of the city usually is where you'll find them. Unfortunately, that means that to move near them, you'll have to pay the highest rents.

The modeling business being what it is guarantees tough competition among modeling agencies for the advertisements. The money to be earned is so stupendous that every agency is vying for a larger and larger slice of the pie. If they weren't aggressive, there wouldn't be any jobs for you or them, and they'd be out looking for other work if they couldn't handle the struggle for power.

It is not really possible to know if you have the type of personality that can cope with all the wheeling and dealing, but it's certainly not a consideration to take lightly unless you are planning to have the one and only agency in an entire area.

STARTING A MODELING SCHOOL

Owning a modeling school could be a great deal of fun, accompanied by equally hard work. Depending on its location, a school could need certification from state boards and from local boards. To find out the requirements in your area, write to your state's capital for that information. A modeling school is also considered a business and thus has to pass certain standards according to the Bureau of Consumer Frauds and Protection and the Better Business Bureau.

In New York State, "dancing, music, pure or fine art, dramatic art" need not be licensed by the state, according to the New York State Education Law, Section 5001. This ruling pertains to New York only and thus should be a consideration for anyone contemplating the opening of a modeling or charm school in New York State. Other states have different requirements.

You have to judge whether the area in which you want to locate will support a school of this nature. In some areas, you might find a mere handful of students, which would necessitate your expanding the school to teaching other curriculum, expanding to include other age groups, or folding. The possibilities all should be carefully weighed before investing a penny. Some sections of the country still do not take any interest in fashion.

After you have tested the waters and found the area to be amenable to the idea of a charm or modeling school, select the location and amount of space accordingly. You may hope to get contracts for advertising from local merchants after you produce a few polished models who could work for them. This bit of confirmation might help you decide if expansion plans could be part of your near future.

What courses will you offer? Can you teach them all yourself? If this is to be a very small enterprise, then you probably can do the instruction.

Finances should be a major consideration. It may take quite a while to get out of the red. Schools can be very successful, but expenses can also be high—rent payment, insurance, telephone bill, receptionist, advertising, textbook (usually one of your own making), electric bill, rental for video equipment, cameras, makeup, faculty (usually professionals in specialized areas), and allotted amounts for guest lecturers to keep the instruction up-to-date. Fashion itself is only that if it is fresh and new.

Publications on fashion around the world also have to be included in the budget. Imported periodicals are very expensive, but they are so important in learning where fashion is established and what each country contributes to the overall look that is created. Exposure to the fashion world should include both imported and domestic publications.

Instructing is very different from modeling, of course. Patience is indispensable, and the desire to help someone else to learn and understand is the priority. If you think that you would enjoy teaching, you could even do some volunteer work in that area. Though it obviously would not be like giving your own courses, it might provide insight into a field that really is not known for its ease. There have been hundreds of masters in their own select fields who not only realized that they were miscast as instructors but also truly hated the teaching end of the professions that they adored as performers.

Give serious thought to the possibility of running a school; then if you still feel that you'd like to try running a school but loathe the instruction part, you could hire instructors and enjoy the administration end of things.

HOW MUCH COULD BE MADE FROM OWNING OR MANAGING A MODELING SCHOOL OR AGENCY?

The smallest agencies in the tiniest towns make the most insignificant incomes in their chosen fields due to a limited clientele and, often, lack of general interest in fashion. When you look into the possibilities of opening a modeling school or agency, look through the past few years of the local Yellow Pages and see how many schools and agencies have not continued to exist in your area. There may be very good reasons *why* the area does not have any modeling establishments. The economy has caused hundreds of these businesses to fold in the past few years. Agencies and schools of modeling that were fairly well established have suddenly disappeared from sight. So thoroughly investigate any area where you think that a modeling business may be just the thing. There is potentially a great deal of money to be earned in the business end of this field. The more clever you are, the better your chances of success.

A modeling agency in a small town could make as little as $20,000, while a modeling school could possibly do the same or better. A medium-sized city would have more people from which to draw both students and clients. For an agency to survive, there have to be both merchants in goodly numbers and models from which the client can choose. The risks are greater and so are the potential profits.

To give you an idea of how an agency makes its money, consider the following: An average model in a medium-sized city is currently making about $15,000 per year. The agency should have at least a few dozen models capable of this income. The agency collects between 20 and 25 percent of their job incomes as its fee. Given all the expenses of running the business of the agency, the money could be pretty tight. Certain areas of our country are still doing a large amount of the entire modeling industry. New York City, Los Angeles, Chicago, Dallas, and a handful of the middle-sized cities are the main hubs. These centers seem to be the better business spots for starting an agency or a school of modeling, although you also encounter greater competition from other existing schools and agencies by locating there.

Several famous models have opened their own agencies in these largest of cities and are doing very well. In fact, many of the most well-known modeling agencies in New York City are owned and run by former models. They are very successful businesswomen and extremely adept managers. Supermodels are rare, but supermodeling agents and their agencies are even more rare. However, you may be that one in millions who has the shrewdness and business sense to start a large agency and keep it afloat.

There are also smaller agencies, specialist agencies, and even an agency run as a franchise. You might want to consider these possibilities, too.

The most popular franchises are the modeling schools, and the income in these would depend greatly on your ability to attract students. There would obviously be better locations than others. These schools are scattered over the fifty states, as required by the population centers. The lowest-paying ownerships or franchises would run around $25,000 per annum, and the largest incomes in owning your own modeling agency would be well up in the millions.

Owning a modeling agency is not everybody's forte. The stress is incredible and the competition deadly. You may want to look into possible related work other than owning or managing a modeling facility, but you are your own best judge. There are very successful agents out there. You may have it in you to be one also!

CHAPTER 10

MODELING'S FUTURE

If current interest is any indication as to the longevity of the profession, then modeling is insured of a brilliant future. Celebrity having been brought into the arena now makes the profession more yearned for than ever. Obsession with youth and beauty has turned models into icons who are adored, are given the royal treatment the world over, and often marry major political or show business powers. Beauty has always been prized, and what can be purchased at great prices fascinates the world press and its followers. It has entertained the masses for centuries to emulate the royal figureheads and often turn them into vapid models, as we have seen happen with most wives of princes or kings. What is worn by these influential ladies is often coveted by the fashionistas. There is now a blur intentionally created by the fashion designers to make society and modeling all and the same. It has certainly succeeded in selling to the masses who so long to be a part of what is happening. Vicariousness is pushing fashion faster than anything else.

There are steadily holding numbers of models continuing to flood the ranks. The agencies are doing well for both themselves and their large rosters of models in *all* areas.

MALE MODELS IN DEMAND

Male modeling also expanded tremendously in the 1990s. The major modeling agencies have all opened divisions for their male models due to the new expanded market. Men are now working as runway models for shows and videos, doing print and live work, and edging into the fashion world that had been dominated exclusively by the female models for decades.

The emergence of the male as an admired figure for his looks alone is a new trend, and the male modeling world is capitalizing on this idea. The male model no longer needs to be a gentleman shown in a size 40 suit as an accessory to an exquisitely turned out high fashion female model, but is more often seen as an entity unto himself. He has the whole gamut of a designer-made wardrobe. Underwear for men has become very status-oriented, and as a result many male models are being hired for their beautiful physiques. This was not the case just a few years ago, when the male model's major purpose was to render a subdued but proper costume, an inspired necessity to any man's wardrobe.

The recent trend toward fashion design in men's apparel has led major newspapers to do extensive sections on menswear from hats to swimwear.

The look that is currently in is one of an unshaven, swarthy sex symbol or blond collegiate-athlete. Unkempt hair and sullen looks now represent a more relaxed overall attitude. The wardrobe of the modern male has expanded to such incredible dimensions that men's cosmetics, fragrances, and facial products are an immense market in themselves. Both live and photographic male models are needed for this ballooning market.

Color is another major change in the men's clothing market. It is not unusual to have the wardrobe include every color of shirt, pants, ties, and jackets that could be imagined. Therefore, the prints and catalogs are now much more extensive than they used to be and are creating more and more work for the male model. The variety of sportswear alone fills pages of ads in magazines, catalogs, newspapers, and on billboards and flyers.

Men's shoes, boots, and sports footwear have become so diversified that they are now classified as fashion also and get lots of prime ad space.

Eyewear has become so chic that men are expected to sport several different kinds of sunglasses, as well as designer frames even if they wear contact lenses.

The high-priced men's clothing market has created thousands of modeling spots. The items are so status-oriented that many are one-of-a-kind. Much male modeling has become prestigious in the same way that female modeling has. Items that were exclusively worn by the super-rich of yesterday are a fast growing market for today's man. Silk pajamas, linen shorts, and cashmere shawl-collared robes that sell for hundreds are fast becoming chic for men.

The well-dressed man of yesterday was more than likely quietly outfitted by his tailor exclusively, and there was no need to advertise style, as it was set by the famous and royal. Today's man is able to dress with much more flair than ever before, and the selection is shown endlessly by the male modeling industry.

It would not be unusual for a male model to make well over $100,000 per year after he started to become established. If he "takes off," his salary could well be over the $150,000 mark. There are men who model the gamut from photographic work to television commercials. They do extremely well at paycheck time and are able to maintain their careers for many years.

Male models are needed very frequently for catalog work. This can be their bread and butter for decades if they are liked by the client and remain attractive. Now some men's clothing does change style dramatically each year, opening another new arena.

Modeling schools accept male models-to-be at age thirteen and upward. This would not be an option in all schools, as some instruct only women. Many schools believe that the male model is mostly interested in television commercials and thus stress that particular area of instruction for men. The television commercial is one of the highest paying areas for the male model, without doubt. The other area where he might stand to make a large amount for one commercial would be in the contract for an exclusive product (similar to that of the Marlboro Man). These are the two that stand alone at the top of the ladder.

A male model could be hired by an agency from about $250.00 to $312.50 per hour as his starting rate. If he becomes popular, his rate increases. An agency will help polish a man into a model if it believes that he has the potential; it will also help with portfolio guidance and with his photographs, making appointments with photographers who may be testing.

The male model today is making his own fashion statement. Ultra high chic at thousand dollar price tags are filling the fashion sections of international papers at an amazing pace. Couture designers are redefining what men should wear when. The tailored suit is no longer the only choice of apparel for an evening out. Everything from a Chanel-motif jacket with matching wool slacks to diamonds-for-him are now *de rigueur.* The most expensive as well as exclusive shops are now catering to the revolutionary new clothing for men. This will surely bode well for the fashion modeling career for many male models, as the advertising and the editorial possibilities are being expanded so greatly.

THE FUTURE OF MODELING FOR WOMEN

Women models have always had the corner on the market, and they are still holding their own in all categories. Women models tend to take advantage of their ability to work in the various markets throughout the world. They also go back and forth when other work, like a television role, is offered. While increases are shown in the number of female models registered, the actual employment of male models has not grown much on an annual basis.

Many women models are branching out into the entire spectrum of modeling possibilities to make as much money as is available while they are employable in the field.

The newest market for the female model is that of video, which is an ever increasing market. The high fashion model is getting much more exposure via video than ever before.

The other area that has opened up expressly for the female model is the area of high fashion with extremely young women showing women's couture (fashion). These young girls are taking over a market that had been solely reserved for women at least ten years older. It has placed a whole different vantage point on the modeling future. If young women of ages eleven to thirteen are to be the representatives of the high fashion market, the prices that they command will fall in the highest ranges. There are contracts offered and signed now that are in the hundreds of thousands for the right look in the preteen years. This trend started about twenty years ago and has taken off. Now all the major agencies are hiring younger and younger girls who would normally be employed by an agency for children's modeling.

Salary rates per hour doubled in some instances between 1990 and now. Catalog work is paying $187.50 per hour at today's pay scale for women. Children now make $125.00 per hour for catalog work. Many female models are now started at pay scales of $1,500.00 per day, and the scale rises with demand for the model!

Women models have more choices today than they have ever had. The increase in salary per hour has been a big step forward, but the opportunity to work in hundreds of different locations has also expanded the viable market. Many young women who would have been limited to working in New York City are working in many major cities in Europe, Scandinavia, Australia, and Japan, as well as in other large cities in the United States.

The market is larger, the work is more varied, and regardless of the immense numbers of men and children who are joining the modeling force, modeling is still the stronghold of a woman's industry. There are many more job opportunities in the modeling field for young women than for any of the other members of the profession. Pretty young women will be in demand to promote the nation's products as long as the American industrial world and a large portion of the advertising industry believe that sexy young women attract both men and women to products.

THE FUTURE OF TELEVISION MODELING

Television modeling is another area that is burgeoning beyond all predictions for making money as a model. There are more possibilities for variety in this medium than in any of the others. The man who is a he-man, wimp, pizza-tosser, or skydiver can make large amounts from television commercials.

For the women models, anything from high fashion to the hands only is possible. All areas for women are soaring. There is no shortage of work in television, but there is end-less competition. Everybody wants a slice of the most well-paying pie.

Male models are making a much more obvious dent in television commercials, as their clothing goes more and more into designer fashions. The men's cosmetic industry is taking off, as is the entire array of leisure items from home computers to sporting gear.

Child models are also doing extremely well, from tiny babies to teenagers. Their field encompasses the major por-tion of the toy market (which is sizable), children's clothing and shoes, medicines for children, and a myriad of other possibilities. In fact the market is so lucrative that many child models are surpassing their counterparts in the adult modeling world. *Everyone loves puppies and babies* is an old adage, but it has paid its weight in gold in the television commercial world. As a case in point, a baby only a few months old made over $13,000 in commercials and their residuals.

The area of television commercials has so expanded that many major modeling agencies that handled basically pho-tographic models have now added separate television divisions to their ranks. Many models used to have the modeling agency do the booking for everything except television commercials; now they are able to have their modeling agent handle the whole market. Agents and managers who do not run modeling agencies also handle television commercial people.

Television has a very solid future and promises many jobs for models of both sexes and the widest variety of ages. The television industry runs on the money of sponsors, and they are in continual need of models to demonstrate their products.

Models and actors used to be looked down upon for doing commercials, but the money and attitudes have both changed noticeably. The biggest names in show business are out there as your stiffest competition for that high-paying commercial.

Billions of dollars are spent annually on commercials for television. That indicates the strength behind the market for the continued need for thousands of television models for future times.

CHAPTER 11

MODELING SCHOOLS AND AGENCIES IN CANADA

Modeling is seeing a tremendous boom in the Canadian marketplace. Vancouver is now being called Hollywood North due to the number of movies being filmed there. Toronto is where it's happening back east. The largest agencies are even handling supermodels. Canada, not unlike the United States, has widely ranging differences in modeling in the smaller towns versus the bigger cities. The tiny areas do have an interest in fashion and modeling and have schools reflecting these needs and commensurate tuitions.

In an outlying area from Toronto, I found that the modeling school offered an eight-week course for $200. The instruction was fairly basic and was given with the lesser-sophisticated girl in mind. Another option for schooling is, of course, to head to the big city first to see what it has to offer. The little area did offer work immediately on the local level, as the school worked as an agent to all the youngsters.

The school in the metropolis started at $1,000 for a thirty-nine hour course that addressed all the ground-laying work such as personal grooming, posing, makeup, and how to present yourself for the neophyte model.

Schools in Canada must meet a carefully registered curriculum set at the government level. They must pass the government's standards to qualify for accreditation.

It is of utmost importance that you check the credentials of the modeling school that you are considering before you pay any tuition. It is quite easy to do this as any accredited school is registered with the Canadian government.

A SAMPLE SCHOOL

All schools will differ somewhat, so this chapter will use one particular school as an example, and variations will be the norm. The modeling curriculum was recently broken down to three categories and sections of classes. The first course is an introduction to modeling through self-awareness. Emphasis is placed on the individual's ideal weight, diet, and exercise. Hair, skin, poise, personality, self-presentation, and etiquette are stressed, as is self-assurance.

Posture, makeup, and wardrobe are detailed for the individual. The age group involved in this curriculum would usually be around thirteen to eighteen for the young women. As this course is basically geared toward the true novice in the modeling world, stress is put on the really basic but professional tricks of the trade. A model must have the capability to "sell" herself, and a client must see a polished, self-assured model if the job is to be hers.

If you are interested in high fashion work, this is the time to discover if you have the real essentials. Everyone can benefit from this introduction course simply to improve their general appearance. However, if you plan to work in the fashion arena of runway and photography, you will probably consider continuation in these courses. You should be between five feet nine inches to six feet tall, well proportioned and square-shouldered, and possess attractive facial features.

The Canadian market does use some shorter models and fuller figures for runway shows at locations like malls, where a more average and heavier woman would be the audience and thus the prospective buyer. Even petite sizes to model junior fashions have some work offers. Specific work through the agency could call for large sizes from 14–20, as well. The type of work would dictate the contents of the school's courses.

Another segment of this particular school offers film workshops for ages thirteen and up. These classes cost $700. Emphasized are the audition, voice, monologue, and scenes using interaction with others. Adapting to the camera is critical for commercial work. Special delivery to the camera is taught. Acting "natural" in front of a camera is more often learned than inherited. Clever acting techniques come into play here to produce a genuine appearance and make a believable situation out of a very artificial one. Videotape is used to allow the student to judge his or her credibility.

The advanced course consists of personal style development by the model. The all important model's bag is detailed so that you will be prepared for all the possibilities that different jobs require. Portfolios and their importance are pinpointed. The Zed card, head shots, and resumes for casting are defined. The ability to handle your finances is critical, as vouchers (how you get paid) will be your own responsibility. A real sense of professionalism is reached in this course, and private attention is given to the individual's strong points and particular talents.

Modeling Classes for Men

The curriculum is not as intricate for men who wish to model. The classes are again grouped into consecutive courses at the particular school chosen as the sample. The basic grooming course is much like that of the women's instruction for the introduction to modeling. The detail for makeup and hairstyle would not be lengthy for the men. The stress for the following courses would be on runway, photographs, films, and video, with all the similar needs used to prepare the women models. Men must learn to sell themselves also, so strong points are brought out by the personal instruction. The entire program for men would run around $700. The course runs for thirteen weeks, three hours at a time on weekdays. There is also a ten-week program for TV acting and commercials. Men involved in the program are reminded that the tuition is tax deductible.

Modeling Classes for Children

The age group for the children's modeling curriculum is from tot to preteen. There are eight two-hour classes wherein the child is taught how to respond to the varied possible situations posed during modeling for photographs, runway, and commercial work. The sample school's tuition is $450. This school is Canadian non-tax exempt. Vocational learning for children is not tax deductible, though children can work and must pay taxes accordingly.

WHERE TO FIND WORK IN CANADA

There are two modeling centers in Canada. The main area for all work is Toronto, where about twenty-five hundred models are currently doing some form of work. The industry has seen tremendous growth in the past years. The most recent modeling center is Vancouver, British Columbia.

Montreal is the other major city for modeling work to be found in Canada. It is estimated that a model who is well established and in demand would be able to command from $75,000 to $100,000 per year.

Work in Montreal would necessitate your having at minimum a basic understanding and command of the French language.

UNIONS

The union for screen acting in Canada is ACTRA. If commercial work is done under this union, the pay scale without voice is $520 and the residual is paid for every thirteen weeks that the commercial is aired. You will need six credits to become a member and only three credits for the same membership if you are an ethnic model, as there is less call for that area in Canada. If you are not a member of ACTRA, the pay scale is usually half of the union wage. Dues are $130 per year plus working dues 1.75 percent of gross income.

BEFORE YOU PROCEED

Several of the Canadian modeling agencies and schools wish to alert potential models who are just starting out to some serious frauds that have left ethical agents quite concerned. They would ask that you approach modeling with a serious eye toward legitimate and honest modeling establishments. If you are a young person, involve your parents, don't answer ads in the paper, and check to make certain that the agency is legitimate or that the school is listed by the Canadian Board of Colleges and Universities. Modeling can be a very rewarding profession, but you will have to be careful not to be naive, as there have been some unpleasant situations due to frauds created by a very few unethical people.

MODELING AGENCIES AND SCHOOLS

Your first step into the modeling world is definitely through an established agency. Set up an interview by phone, fax, or in person, and then be at that appointment on time! Listen to everything the agent has to offer, and then ask any questions you may have. The professional eye of the agent will critique you while you are there. Try to remain calm and relaxed under this scrutiny. After all, he or she must assess your salability and profitability during this short interview. If you don't fit in, there is no future for either of you.

There is no salary in modeling, only commissions to be made on the actual jobs, so an honest guess is the best an agent can give you. Every detail should be carefully addressed, and unless you have an excellent memory, you'll want to take notes. A positive and professional attitude is your best door opener. If you are late or careless in your personal appearance or hygiene, you will certainly be ushered out the door and considered a waste of time.

Open call is the fastest way to a modeling interview. All the big agencies have these events, and it is the proverbial cattle call. Thousands of wanna-be models pour into the agency armed with head-shots and hopes. The statistics are really amazing in that only one in a thousand is offered a call back!

If you are among those selected few, give serious consideration to all the details covered in the interview before you sign a contract. You may want to look at several agencies or have an attorney look at what you are signing if you don't understand the legalese. Many a supermodel has a financial manager who can negotiate those huge contracts into even more astronomical fees.

A PARTIAL LIST OF AGENCIES AND SCHOOLS IN THE UNITED STATES AND CANADA

An *A* after name indicates *agency;* an *S* indicates *school.*

Alabama

Birmingham

Real People Models & Talent, Inc. (A)
714 Thirty-Second Street
Birmingham, AL 35233

Alaska

Anchorage

John Robert Powers (A, S)
300 E. Dimond Boulevard
Anchorage, AK 99515

Arizona

Phoenix

Signature Models & Talent (A)
2600 N. Forty-Fourth Street,
Suite 209
Phoenix, AZ 85008

Scottsdale

Elizabeth Savage Talent (A)
4949 East Lincoln Drive
Scottsdale, AZ 85253

California

Beverly Hills

William Morris Agency (A)
151 El Camino Drive
Beverly Hills, CA 90212

La Jolla

Jet Set Management &
Agency (A)
7855 Fay Avenue #350
La Jolla, CA 92037

Noveau Model & Talent
Management, Inc. (A)
909 Prospect Street, Suite 230
La Jolla, CA 92037

Long Beach

Chic Models (A)
236 Quincy Avenue
Long Beach, CA 90803

Los Alamedes

Barbizon Agency (A)
4281 Katella Avenue
Los Alamedes, CA 90720

Los Angeles

CHN International Agency (A)
7428 Santa Monica Boulevard
Los Angeles, CA 90046

C'la Vie Model (A)
7507 Sunset Boulevard
- Los Angeles, CA 90046

San Diego

San Diego Model Management (A)
824 Camino Del Rio N, Suite
552
San Diego, CA 92108

San Francisco

City Model Management (A)
123 Townsend Street, Suite
510
San Francisco, CA 94107

Look Model Agency (A)
166 Geary Street
San Francisco, CA 94108

Top Models & Talent (A)
870 Market Street, Suite 1076
San Francisco, CA 94102

Colorado

Colorado Springs

Bella Models (A)
4255 Bardot Drive
Colorado Springs, CO 80920

Denver

John Casablancas (A)
7600 E. Eastman Avenue
Denver, CO 80231

Connecticut

Stamford

Barbizon Agency (A)
1051 Long Ridge Road
Stamford, CT 06903

Florida

Fort Lauderdale

Model & Talent Agency (A)
2810 East Oakland Park
Boulevard
Fort Lauderdale, FL 33306

Jaques Models, Inc. (A)
2440 E. Commercial Boulevard
Fort Lauderdale, FL 33308

John Casablancas (A)
3343 W. Commercial
Boulevard
Fort Lauderdale, FL 33306

Models Exchange (A)
2425 E. Commercial
Boulevard
Fort Lauderdale, FL 33308

Miami

Boss Models-Miami (A)
539A Euclid Avenue
Miami Beach, FL 33139

Ford Models (A)
826 Ocean Drive
Miami Beach, FL 33139

John Casablancas (A)
10491 N. Kendall Drive
Miami, FL 33176

Pembroke Pines
Barbizon School of Modeling
(S)
8385 Pines Boulevard
Pembroke Pines, FL 33024

Tampa

John Casablancas Modeling &
Career Center (S, A)
5215 Laurel W.
Tampa, FL 33607

On Location Model & Talent (A)
1211 N. Westshore Boulevard
Tampa, FL 33607

Trends Model Talent, Inc. (A)
2900 Seventh Avenue
Tampa, FL 33605

Winter Park

John Casablancas (A)
329 Park Avenue S.
Winter Park, FL 32789

Lisa Maile Image Modeling &
Acting (A)
999 South Orlando Avenue
Winter Park, FL 32789

Georgia

Atlanta

Arlene Wilson Model
Management (A)
887 West Marietta Street NW
Atlanta, GA 30318

Bauder Fashion College (S)
Phipps Plaza
3500 Peachtree Road N.E.
Atlanta, GA 30326

Hawaii

Honolulu

John Robert Powers (A)
1314 S. King Street
Honolulu, HI 96814

Illinois

Chicago

Barbizon of Chicago (S)
541 N. Fairbanks
Chicago, IL 60611

David & Lee Model
Management (A)
70 W. Hubbard Street
Chicago, IL 60610

Elite Model Management (A)
    212 W. Superior Street
    Chicago, IL 60610

ETA, Inc. (A)
    7588 S. Chicago Avenue
    Chicago, IL 60619

Geddes Agency (A)
    1633 N. Halsted Street
    Chicago, IL 60614

John Robert Powers (S)
    27 E. Monroe Street
    Chicago, IL 60603

Shirley Hamilton Inc. (A)
    333 E. Ontario Street
    Chicago, IL 60611

Stewart Talent Agency (A)
    212 W. Superior Street
    Chicago, IL 60610

Indiana

Evansville

Beau Madame (A)
    521 N. Green River Road
    Evansville, IN 47715

Joyce's Stars of Tomorrow (A)
    2205 E. Morgan
    Evansville, IN 47715

Fort Wayne

Charmaine School & Model
    Agency (A)
    3538 Stellhorn Road
    Fort Wayne, IN 46815

Hobart

Evelyn Lahaie Modeling
    & Talent (A)
    P.O. #614
    Hobart, IN 46342

Indianapolis

Union Street Modeling & Talent
    Agency (A)
    One Virginia Avenue
    P.O. Box 2345
    Indianapolis, IN 46206

Mishawaka

AAA Modeling & Talent Agency
    (S, A)
    736 E. Tenth Place
    Mishawaka, IN 46544

Iowa

Cedar Rapids

Elan Training & Talent (A)
    223 Lenora Drive NW
    Cedar Rapids, IA 52405

The Image Group (A)
    417 First Avenue
    Cedar Rapids, IA 52401

Des Moines

Avant Studios, Inc. (A)
    7600 University
    Des Moines, IA 50325

Kansas

Kansas City

Career Images Model & Talent
    Agency (A)
    8519 Lathrop Avenue
    Kansas City, KS 66109

Wichita

Focus Model Management (A)
    155 North Market
    Wichita, KS 67202

Kentucky

Louisville

Alix Adams Model School &
    Agency (S, A)
    9813 Merioneth Drive
    Louisville, KY 40299

Madisonville

Cosmo Model & Talent Agency
    (A)
    1083 N. Main Street
    Madisonville, KY 42431

Louisiana

New Orleans

About Faces Model & Talent
    Management (A)
    201 Charles Avenue
    New Orleans, LA 70170

New Orleans Model/Talent
    Agency (A)
    1347 Magazine Street
    New Orleans, LA 70130

Maryland

Baltimore

Nova Models, Inc. (A)
    206 N. Liberty Street
    Baltimore, MD 21201

Ramp Model Management (A)
    403 N. Charles Street
    Baltimore, MD 21201

Massachusetts

Boston

Barbizon Agency (A)
    607 Boylston Street
    Boston, MA 02116

Cameo Kids Modeling & Talent
    Agency (A)
    437 Boylston Street
    Boston, MA 02116

John Robert Powers Career
    School (S)
    175 Andover Street
    Denvers, MA 01923

Maggie, Inc. (A)
    35 Newbury Street
    Boston, MA 02116

The Model's Group
    164 Newbury Street
    Boston, MA 02116

Modeling Career Concepts (A)
    374 Congress Street
    Boston, MA 02210

Worcester

John Robert Powers
    390 Main Street
    Worcester, MA 01608

Michigan

Grand Rapids

Pastiche Models & Talent,
    Inc. (A)
    1514 Wealthy Street SE, Suite
    292
    Grand Rapids, MI 49506

Unique Models & Talent (A)
    4485 Plainfield NE
    Grand Rapids, MI 49505

Lansing

Adams' Pro Modeling &
    Finishing School (A, S)
    2722 E. Michigan
    Lansing, MI 48912

Class Modeling/Talent Agency
    (A)
    2722 E. Michigan
    Lansing, MI 48912

Plymouth

John Casablancas Modeling &
        Career Center
    44450 Pinetree Drive
    Plymouth, MI 48170

Southfield

Milane Modeling (A)
    29425 Northwestern Highway
    Suite 100
    Southfield, MI 48034

Sterling Heights

John Casablancas
    38700 Van Dyke Avenue
    Sterling Heights, MI 48312

New York

Buffalo

June II Model Agency (A)
    143 Allen Street
    Buffalo, NY 14202

L Models
    1807 Elmwood Avenue
    Buffalo, NY 14207

New York City

Barbizon Modeling Agency
    (S, A)
    15 Penn Plaza
    New York, NY 10001

Bethann Management Co., Inc.
    (A)
    36 N. Moore
    New York, NY 10013

Boss Models, Inc. (A)
    1 Gansvoort
    New York, NY 10013

Classique Model Agency (A)
    29 E. Tenth Street
    New York, NY 10003

Click Model Management (A)
    881 Seventh Avenue
    New York, NY 10019

Eastwood Talent Corp. (A)
    44 W. Twenty-Fourth Street
    New York, NY 10011

Elite Model Management Corp.
    (A)
    111 E. Twenty-Second Street
    New York, NY 10010

Elite Runway Inc. (A)
    149 Madison Avenue
    New York, NY 10022

Elizabeth Associates Inc. (A)
    129 East Thirty-Ninth Street
    New York, NY 10016

Ellen Harth, Inc. (A)
    149 Madison Avenue
    New York, NY 10022

Flaunt Model Management Inc.
    (A)
    114 East Thirty-Second Street
    New York, NY 10013

Ford Models (Men & Women) (A)
142 Greene Street
New York, NY 10012

Ford Model Agency (A)
344 E. Fifty-Ninth Street
New York, NY 10022

Gilla Roos Ltd. (A)
16 W. Twenty-Second Street
New York, NY 10010

International Beautiful People
Unlimited Inc. (A)
1841 Broadway
New York, NY 10023

J & R Studio (A)
170 Varick Street
New York, NY 10012

Jade International (A)
1534 Third Avenue
New York, NY 10016

Kids Power (A)
161 West Sixteenth Street
New York, NY 10010

Marge McDermott Enterprises
Agency (A)
216 E. Thirty-Ninth Street
New York, NY 10016

McDonald/Richards, Inc. (A)
156 Fifth Avenue
New York, NY 10010

Modeling Association
of America International
Inc.
350 E. Fifty-Fourth Street
New York, NY 10022

Models Guild
265 W. Fourteenth Street
New York, NY 10010

Models Mart Ltd.
42 W. Thirty-Eighth Street
New York, NY 10018

Models Service Agency (A)
570 Seventh Avenue
New York, NY 10018

Nytro Inc.
134 Spring Street
New York, NY 10012

Ophelia De Vore (S)
350 Fifth Avenue
New York, NY 10118

Plus Models (A)
49 W. Thirty-Seventh
Street
New York, NY 10018

Van Der Veer Models (A)
400 E. Fifty-Seventh Street
New York, NY 10022

Wilhelmina Models Inc. (A)
300 Park Avenue South
New York, NY 10016

Zoli Management Inc. (A)
3 West Eighteenth Street
New York, NY 10011

North Carolina

Asheboro

The Nancy Watson Agency (A)
17 N. Oak Forest Drive
Asheboro, NC 27203

Charlotte

John Casablancas Modeling &
      Career Center
   830 Tyvola Road
   Charlotte, NC 20217

Raleigh

Esteem Model & Talent
      Management (A)
   3820 Merton Drive
   Raleigh, NC 27609

Ohio

Akron

Protocol Model & Talent Agency
      (A)
   1969 N. Cleveland-Massilon
      Road
   Akron, OH 44333

Cleveland

Barbizon School & Agency (A, S)
   6450 Rockside Woods
   Cleveland, OH 44131

David & Lee Inc. (A)
   1300 E. Ninth Street
   Bond Court Building
   Cleveland, OH 44114

Mélange (A)
   3130 Mayfield Road
   Cleveland Heights, OH 44118

Stone Model & Talent Agency (A)
   6450 Rockslide Woods, LL#2
   Cleveland, OH 44131

Taxi Model Management (A)
   1300 West Seventy-Eighth
   Cleveland, OH 44102

Tommye's New Attitude (A)
   3713 Lee Road
   Cleveland, OH 44120

Columbus

Cline and Mosic Talent Agency,
      Inc. (A)
   1350 W. Fifth Avenue
   Columbus, OH 43212

Creative Talent Co. (A)
   1102 Neil Avenue
   Columbus, OH 43201

Elite Faces, Inc—Real Faces (A)
   1415 E. Dublin-Granville Road
   Columbus, OH 43229

Go International Model
      Management (A)
   1227 Pennsylvania Avenue
   Columbus, OH 43201

Jeanette Grider School of
      Modeling (S)
   1453 East Main Street
   Columbus, OH 43205

L'Esprit Models & Talent Inc. (A)
   2151 E. Dublin-Granville Road
   Columbus, OH 43229

Noni Agency (A) (S)
   172 E. State Street
   Columbus, OH 43215

John Casablancas (A)
  6322 Busch Boulevard
  Columbus, OH 43229

John Robert Powers School &
    Agency (S, A)
  5900 Roche Drive, Suite 205
  Columbus, OH 43229

Dayton

Bette Massie Inc. (A)
  8075 McEwen Road
  Dayton, OH 45458

Creative Talent Network (A)
  10019 Paragon Road
  Dayton, OH 45458

Sharkey Agency Inc. (A, S)
  1299 Lyons Road
  Dayton, OH 45458

Pennsylvania

Philadelphia

Creative Source Management (A)
  5510 Greene Street
  Philadelphia, PA 19144

Expressions Agency (A)
  110 Church Street
  Philadelphia, PA 91906

John Robert Powers (S)
  1528 Spruce Street
  Philadelphia, PA 19102

Reinhard Model & Talent Agency
    (A)
  2021 Arch Street
  Philadelphia, PA 19103

Pittsburgh

Barbizon School of Modeling (S)
  9 Parkway Center, Suite 160
  Pittsburgh, PA 15205

John Casablancas (A)
  2020 Ardmore Boulevard
  Pittsburgh, PA 15221

Van Enterprises
  9600 Perry Highway
  Pittsburgh, PA 15237

Reading

Donatelli Modeling & Casting
    Agency (A)
  156 Madison Avenue, Hyde
    Park
  Reading, PA 19605

Rhode Island

Providence

Debi Cusick D'Iorio
  1085 Chalkstone Avenue
  Providence, RI 02904

Warwick

Character Kids (A)
  1692 Warwick Avenue
  Warwick, RI 02889

John Casablancas (A)
  One Lambert Lind Highway
  Warwick, RI 02888

South Carolina

Columbia

Collins Models-Studio & Agency
  1441 Greenhill Road
  Columbia, SC 29206

Jenny Trussell Modeling & Talent
    Agency (A)
    1030 St. Andrews Road
    Columbia, SC 29210

Millie Lewis Model & Talent
    Agency (A)
    3612 Landmark Drive
    Columbia, SC 29206

Russell Adair Fashion Studio (A)
    1112 Meeting Street
    West Columbia, SC 29169

Tennessee

Chattanooga

Ambiance Modeling Agency
    (A)(S)
    5959 Shallow Ford Road
    Chattanooga, TN 37402

Knoxville

Barbizon School of Modeling (S)
    408 N. Cedar Bluff Road
    Knoxville, TN 37923

Model & Talent Access (A)
    109 North Shore Drive
    Knoxville, TN 37919

Talent Trek Agency (A)
    406 Eleventh Street
    Knoxville, TN 37916

Memphis

Donna's School of Modeling (S)
    4294 Stage Road
    Memphis, TN 38128

Elite Artists Inc. (A)
    785 Crossover Lane
    Memphis, TN 38117

John Robert Powers Modeling
    and Career School (S)
    5118 Park Avenue
    Memphis, TN 38117

Texas

Austin

Acclaim (A)
    4107 Med. Pky., #210
    Austin, TX 78756

Class (A)
    3603 Southridge Drive
    Austin, TX 78704

K. Hall Model & Talent (A)
    101 W. Sixth Street
    Austin, TX 78701

Dallas

Barbizon School of Modeling
    (A, S)
    12700 Hillcrest Road
    Dallas, TX 75230

Clipse Model & Talent
    Management (A)
    3301 McKinney Avenue, #200
    Dallas, TX 75204

Dallas Model Group (A)
    12700 Hillcrest Road
    Dallas, TX 75230

Elan Model & Talent
    Management (A)
    4211 McEwen Road
    Dallas, TX 75244

John Robert Powers Modeling (S)
    13601 Preston Road
    Dallas, TX 75240

K D Studios (S)
2600 Stemmons Freeway
Dallas, TX 75207

Margo Manning Casting &
Acting Studio (S)(A)
6360 Lyndon B. Johnson
Freeway
Dallas, TX 75240

Page Parkes Models Rep (A)
3131 McKinney Avenue
Dallas, TX 75204

Stars Over Texas
John Carpenter Freeway
Dallas, TX 75247

Tanya Blair-Tiba Inc. (A)
4528 McKinney Avenue
Dallas, TX 75205

El Paso

Fran Simon Talent & Modeling
9619 Acer Avenue
El Paso, TX 79925

Mannequin Manor Fashion
Career School (S)
9611 Acer Avenue
El Paso, TX 79925

Houston

Actors & Models of Houston
Agency (A)
7887 San Felipe Street
Houston, TX 77063

Barbizon
621 Wellesley Drive
Houston, TX 77024

Elite Productions (A)
11909 Dunlap Street
Houston, TX 77035

First Models & Talent Agency (A)
5433 Westheimer Road, #305
Houston, TX 77056

Hamil Neal Agency Inc. (A)
7887 San Felipe
Houston, TX 77063

Mayo-Hill School of Modeling
(S)
7887 San Felipe Street, #127
Houston, TX 77063

Page Parkes School of Modeling
(S)
5353 W. Alabama Street
Houston, TX 77056

Virginia

McLean

The Erickson Agency (A)
1491 Chain Bridge Road
McLean, VA 22101

Washington

Seattle

Carol James Talent Agency (A)
117 South Main
Seattle, WA 98104

Edge Model Management (A)
911 E. Pike
Seattle, WA 98122

Kids Team (A)
911 E. Pike
Seattle, WA 98122

Seattle Models Guild
    1807 Seventh
    Seattle, WA 98101

TCM Models (A)
    2200 Sixth Avenue
    Seattle, WA 98121

Washington, DC

Anne Schwab's Model Store
    1529 Wisconsin Avenue
    Washington, DC 20007

The Artist Agency
    3068 M Street NW
    Washington, DC 20007

Central Casting Inc. (A)
    623 Pennsylvania Avenue SE
    Washington, DC 20003

Stars Casting(A)
    1301 Twentieth Street NW
    Washington, DC 20036

Canada

Brampton

Bickerton Models (A)
    499 Main Street
    Brampton, ONT

Mississauga

Barbizon
    1590 Dundas E.
    Mississauga, ONT

Montreal

Folio Montreal (A)
    295 de la Commune Ovest
    Montreal, QB H2Y 21E

Thunder Bay

Modelling Association of Canada
    176 Rupert Street
    Thunder Bay, ONT

Toronto

The Armstrong Group (A)
    78 Berkeley Street
    Toronto, ONT

Bickerton Models (A)
    499 Main Street
    Toronto, ONT

Bookings EMEL
        Management (A)
    106 Front E.
    Toronto, ONT

Carolyn's Modelling & Self
        Improvement Agency (A)
    16 Britannia Road E.
    Toronto, ONT

Elite Models (A)
    119 Spadina Avenue
    Toronto, ONT

Kool Kids (A)
    25 Imperial Street
    Toronto, ONT

Mannequin Model & Talent
        Agency Inc. (S)
    1251 Yonge
    Toronto, ONT

Nexxt Model Inc. (A)
    2200 Yonge
    Toronto, ONT

Nina G. Model & Talent
    Agencies Inc.
  114 Cumberland
  Toronto, ONT

Reinhart-Perkins Modelling &
    Talent Agency (A)
  2120 Queen E.
  Toronto, ONT

Silver Screen Talent Group (A)
  28 Atlantic
  Toronto, ONT

Sutherland Models (S)
  20 Eglinton E.
  Toronto, ONT

TELEVISION COMMERCIAL AGENTS

New York City

Actor Reps of New York
  1501 Broadway
  New York, NY 10019

Agency for the Performing
    Arts, Inc.
  888 Seventh Avenue
  New York, NY 10022

American Model Management
    Corp.
  155 Spring Street
  New York, NY 10012

Elite Model Management
    Corp.
  111 E. Twenty-Second
    Street
  New York, NY 10010

Ford Models Inc.
  344 E. Fifty-Ninth Street
  New York, NY 10022

McDonald/Richards, Inc.
  156 Fifth Avenue
  New York, NY 10010

Models & Talent Management
  415 Seventh Avenue
  New York, NY 10001

Wilhelmina Models Inc.
  300 Park Avenue South
  New York, NY 10016

William Morris Agency,
    Inc.
  1325 Sixth Avenue
  New York, NY 10019

Zoli Models Inc.
  3 West Eighteenth
    Street
  New York, NY 10011

California

Los Angeles

Nina Blanchard Agency
  957 Cole Avenue
  Los Angeles, CA 90028

William Morris
  151 El Camino Drive
  Beverly Hills, CA 90212

San Francisco

Brebner Agencies Inc.
  China Basin Building
  Suite 144
  185 Berry Street
  San Francisco, CA 94123

Dorie Model And Talent Agency
  2421 Lombard
  San Francisco, CA 94123

PUBLICATIONS FOR MODELS

AMERICAN PERIODICALS

Elle Publishing
   1633 Broadway
   New York, NY 10019

Glamour
   350 Madison Avenue
   New York, NY 10017

Harpers Bazaar
   1700 Broadway
   New York, NY 10019

Seventeen Magazine
   850 Third Avenue
   New York, NY 10022

Teen Magazine
   437 Madison Avenue
   New York, NY 10022

Vogue Magazine
   350 Madison Avenue
   New York, NY 10022

FOREIGN PERIODICALS

Elle
   E.D.I., 7 (F.E.P. Hachette et
      Cie.) S.N.C.
   Locataire-gerant
   6 Rue Ancelle
   92525 Neuilly-Sur-Seine,
      France

Vogue
   4 Place du Palais-Bourbon
   75007 Paris, France

Marie Clair
   11 Bis, Rue Boissy-d'Anglais
   75008 Paris, France

NEWSPAPERS TO THE TRADE

BackStage
   Back Stage Publications
   1515 Broadway
   New York, NY 10036

Back Stage
   2035 Westwood
      Boulevard, #210
   Los Angeles, CA 90025

Show Business
   1501 Broadway
   New York, NY 10036

Variety Inc.
   245 W. Seventeenth Street
   New York, NY 10011

Womens Wear Daily
   7 W. Thirty-Fourth Street
   New York, NY 10018

APPENDIX D

BIBLIOGRAPHY OF
RELATED READING

Aucoin, Kevin. *Making Faces.* Foreword by Gene Rowlands. New York: Little Brown and Company, 1997.

Cox, Janice. *Natural Beauty for All Seasons.* New York: Henry Holt & Co., 1996.

Crawford, Cindy, Sonia Kashuk, and Kathleen Boyes. *Cindy Crawford's Basic Face.* New York: Broadway Books, 1996.

Davis, Julie. *Young Skin for Life.* Emmaus, PA: Rodale Press, Inc., 1995.

De Castelbajac, Kate. *The Face of the Century.* New York: Rizzoli, 1995.

Denwald, Richard & Anthony Chiappone. *For Men Only: Secrets of a Successful Image.* Amherst, NY: Prometheus Books, 1995.

Fried, Stephen. *Thing of Beauty.* New York: Pocket Books, a division of Simon & Schuster Inc., 1993.

Gross, Kim Johnson, Jeff Stone, text by Rachel Urquhart. *Woman's Face.* New York: Copyright by Chic Simple, LLC. Alfred A. Knopf, Inc., 1997.

Gross, Michael. *Model: The Ugly Business of Beautiful Women.* New York: William Morrow and Company, Inc., 1995.

Hartman, Toni. *Fabulous You.* New York: Berkley Books, The Berkley Publishing Group, 1995.

Irons, Diane. *The World's Best-Kept Beauty Secrets.* Naperville, IL: Sourcebooks, Inc. 1997.

Morris, Sandra. *The Model Manual.* London: The Orion Publishing Group, 1997.

Widdows, Lee. *Catwalk: Working with Models.* London: Batsford, 1996.